646·7

PST

Short loan.

Principles and Techniques for the Electrologist

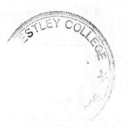

D0230762

Also published by Stanley Thornes (Publishers) Ltd:

Ann Gallant	*Principles and Techniques for the Beauty Specialist*
Ann Gallant	*Body Treatments and Dietetics for the Beauty Therapist*
W E Arnould-Taylor	*The Principles and Practice of Physical Therapy*
W E Arnould-Taylor	*A Textbook of Anatomy and Physiology*
W E Arnould-Taylor	*A Textbook of Holistic Aromatherapy*
Ann Hagman	*The Aestheticienne—Simple Theory and Practice*
Ann Hagman	*Aesthetics for the Therapist*
Janet Simms	*A Practical Guide to Beauty Therapy*

Principles and Techniques for the Electrologist

Ann Gallant

F.S.H.B.Th., Int.B.Th.Dip., DRE (Tutor)

Formerly Lecturer Responsible
for Beauty Therapy at
Chichester College of Further Education and
Gloucestershire College of Arts and Technology

Stanley Thornes (Publishers) Ltd

© text Ann Gallant 1983

© diagrams Stanley Thornes (Publishers) Ltd 1983

All rights reserved. No part of this publication may be
reproduced or transmitted in any form or by any means,
electronic or mechanical, including photocopy, recording, or
any information storage and retrieval system, without
permission in writing from the publisher or under licence from
the Copyright Licensing Agency Limited. Further details of
such licences (for reprographic reproduction) may be obtained
from the Copyright Licensing Agency Limited, of 90 Tottenham
Court Road, London W1P 9HE.

First published 1983 by
Stanley Thornes (Publishers) Ltd
Ellenborough House
Wellington Street
CHELTENHAM GL50 1YD

00 / 10

British Library Cataloguing in Publication Data

Gallant, Ann
    Principles and techniques for the electrologist
    1. Hair—Removal   2. Electrolysis
    I. Title
    646.7'24   RL115.5

    ISBN 0–85950–489–1

Phototypeset by
Tradespools Limited, Frome, Somerset
Printed and bound in Great Britain at
Redwood Books, Trowbridge, Wiltshire.

To my husband Rob who helped me in so many ways to complete this book and make it possible, and to my friend and teacher, Frances Godfrey DRE, whose example, knowledge and encouragement gave me my love of electrology, which resulted in this book for the profession.

Contents

Preface

A need has existed for a long time for a book on both the practical techniques and theory relating to electrology—permanent hair removal by short wave diathermy. *Principles and Techniques for the Electrologist* fills this need and provides practically biased information on the operating techniques needed to become skilled in the difficult task of permanent hair removal using the epilation method. Background theory relating to the advisability, efficiency and safety of the treatment has been integrated throughout the book, to stress the inter-relationship between theory and practice that is necessary to ensure overall success in the work.

Information has been provided on the endocrine system, to give readers an awareness of the relationship of unwanted hair growth to the physical state of the individual. This knowledge, reinforced by study of individual case histories, will help to guide operators in their treatment application, and provides a broader view of the field of study. Students and practitioners alike will find it a useful companion and guide in their worthwhile and exacting work.

ANN GALLANT

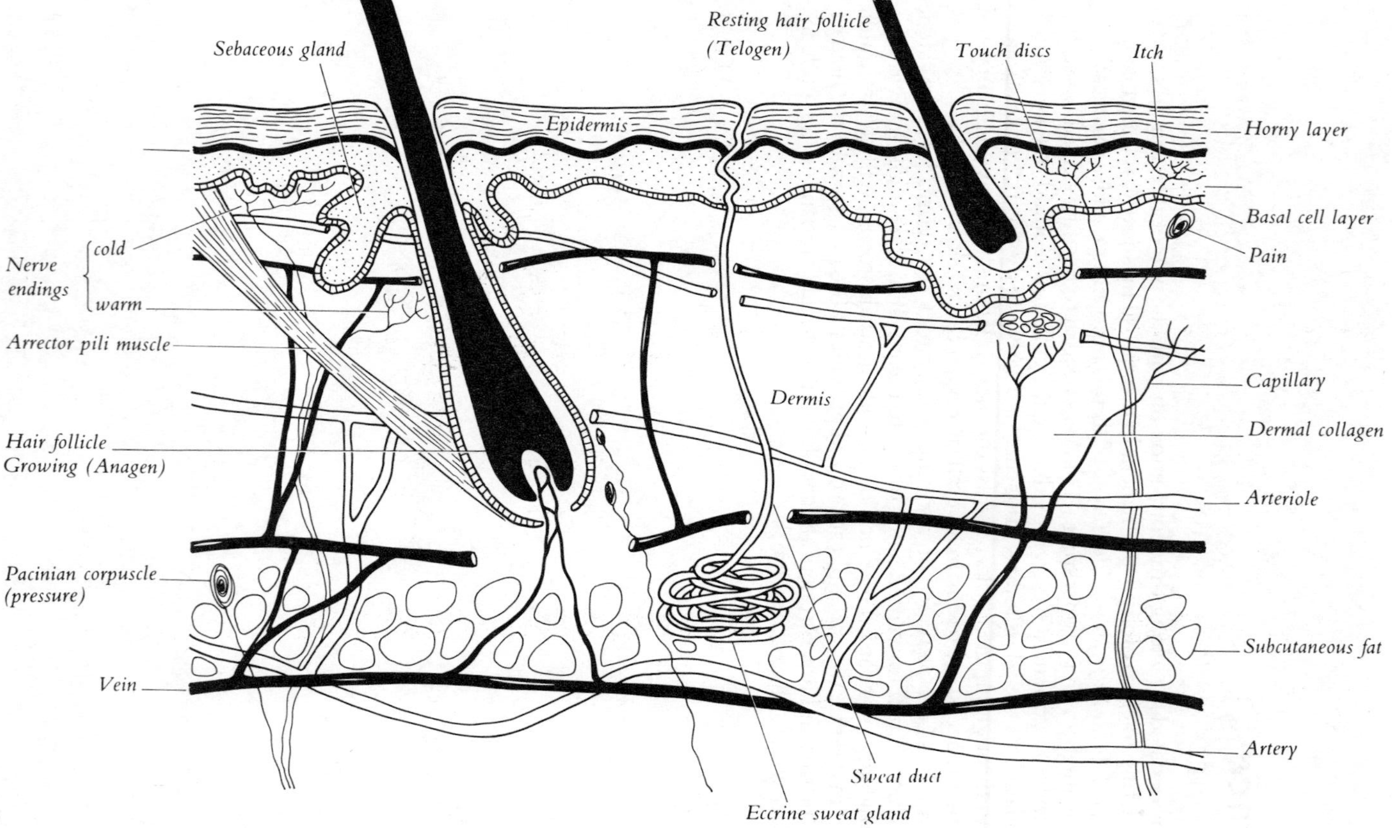

Horny layer

Basal cell layer

Pain

Itch

Capillary

Dermal collagen

Arteriole

Subcutaneous fat

Artery

Touch discs

Resting hair follicle (Telogen)

Epidermis

Dermis

Sweat duct

Eccrine sweat gland

Sebaceous gland

Nerve endings {cold, warm}

Arrector pili muscle

Hair follicle Growing (Anagen)

Pacinian corpuscle (pressure)

Vein

SKIN DIAGRAM

Chapter 1

Introduction to Permanent Hair Removal

The work of the electrologist embraces all forms of permanent hair removal and provides a worthwhile and rewarding service to the public—a service for which there appears to be an ever increasing need. Electrology is an intricate process requiring skill, patience, sympathy and a sound knowledge of background factors to ensure success. In order to offer a permanent solution to the distressing problem of unwanted, superfluous hair growth, the operator must combine practical expertise with a theoretical understanding of the underlying physical factors which influence the growth and behaviour of the hair follicles.

The task facing the electrologist is to destroy the hair growth without damaging the skin or altering its texture or appearance. This is accomplished by introducing a destructive force to the active reproductive area of the follicle, usually by means of a fine, metal needle probe, so that damage is confined to the area where it is specifically needed. The discharge of energy into the moist bulb area of the hair at the base of the follicle ensures maximum destruction and limits associated skin damage in surrounding tissues. This results not only in the removal of the 'dead' hair giving the client an immediate improvement in appearance, but also in the destruction or reduction of the follicle's capacity to regenerate new hair.

Several methods of permanent hair removal are currently available. These are known to the general public as **electrolysis**, a term which, although not strictly accurate, serves to inform the public of the service available. **Epilation** is the method most widely used, providing excellent results quickly and with minimal skin disruption during treatment. It is the removal of hair by *short wave diathermy*—a treatment with electric current which generates heat causing coagulation and eventual destruction of the active hair-producing area of the follicle. Also still available is the **electrolysis** method itself based on the use of galvanic current to produce a chemical reaction in the skin. In its original form it pioneered permanent hair removal in the 1940s and established the word 'electrolysis' firmly in the public's mind as representing *permanent* hair removal. Now improved almost beyond recognition in terms of its application, the basic principles of chemical destruction remain valid and are a useful alternative for permanent removal in some instances of difficult or stubborn hair growth.

An understanding of how hairs are structured in the skin, and how their growth and behaviour are altered by hormones is vital for success. The cause of the client's hair problem, its background and its likely pattern of development, provide guidelines as to the best treatment solution. This knowledge, when linked with a careful assessment of the client's capacity for electrology, provides the best method and timing of treatments aimed at achieving maximum success.

Most hair growth problems presented for treatment are *cosmetic* in nature, that is they are not considered to be directly related to illness or a change in the individual's physical condition. The problem may be linked to a family or racial tendency to hairiness, but the client may only seek treatment if the condition becomes excessive or the hair growth is abnormal in its position on the body. More commonly, the problem is a result of normal hormonal changes in the body which cause increased activity of the follicles, thus altering fine hair growth into a visible and distressing superfluous hair problem. The fine downy hairs of the facial area seem especially sensitive to these minute hormonal changes. The stages of life where hormonal activity increases or alters, such as puberty, pregnancy and the menopause, are the most susceptible for hair growth problems.

All hair growth, whether a problem or not, is influenced by hormones and responds to internal messages transmitted via the blood stream. An understanding of the relationship between the endocrine system, which controls hormonal levels in the body, and the hair follicle and its growth, is essential to the electrologist, not only to promote successful treatment but also to indicate those conditions which would benefit from medical attention. In a small proportion of cases the unwanted hair growth may be directly associated with an *abnormal hormonal imbalance* in the body, or a change in the physical health of the individual. It may be as a direct result of illness, since changes in the skin and hair growth are some of the first indications of an abnormality. Whatever the cause, the electrologist has a responsibility to refer her clients for medical attention whenever it would seem advantageous. Remedial work, performed in conjunction with medical treatment, is particularly rewarding as the clients derive both physical and psychological benefit from the electrologist's work.

Balanced against the electrologist's knowledge of the condition and her ability to perform the techniques of treatment, is her skill in handling the client in a sympathetic and professional manner. Judgement of the client's capacity for treatment, both in terms of her skin condition and temperament, is important as it provides the guidelines for the planning of treatment. Excessive hair growth, low tolerance of discomfort or poor skin-healing problems all affect the manner in which the treatment is applied and also the timetable for treatment. Although a permanent solution to the hair problem is the major aim, the way in which this may be achieved can vary greatly.

Building up a client's confidence and trust helps to reduce anxiety and discomfort and improves co-operation in the treatment plan. The rapport which can develop over extended periods of treatment supports the client through difficult periods of the programme, when spirits are low and a solution seems far away. It ensures that the client perseveres and does not give up in despair at a critical stage of improvement—for in difficult cases, treatment can be lengthy, even with the most expert of techniques, the latest equipment and the back-up of medical expertise.

The electrologist can become *technically expert* through practice and observation of a wide range of hair and skin conditions; by development of a *sense of touch* she will increase accuracy and minimize discomfort for the client, thus allowing more work to be accomplished with less harmful skin effects, and so bringing the treatment to a successful conclusion more rapidly.

It is likely that, with scientific and medical advances, methods of treating unwanted hair will change in the future and it is to be hoped that professional electrologists will contribute to these advances from their experience. Any system which produces permanent results, while reducing the pain element and associated skin damage, will be welcomed. Improvements will doubtless concentrate on making the treatment simpler to apply and control, so bringing faster results. When an easier system emerges which is *safe* and *effective*, it will become part of professional electrology.

Electrologists have the opportunity to advance and reinforce the valuable work accomplished by the pioneers of permanent hair removal, whose efforts have won electrology public acceptance and medical recognition for its value in improving the morale of those individuals disfigured by superfluous hair. Electrology is now an accepted and respected field of activity, but, mainly because of anxiety surrounding the application and worry over scarring, there still remains a large untapped market for professional work.

By her skill and the maintenance of high professional standards, the electrologist should work to ensure that all individuals who require and seek permanent hair removal can receive it from a well-qualified and caring practitioner—one who supports and is bound by ethical standards of work and behaviour.

The aim of this book is to give the operator confidence in her skills, and to provide her with the information necessary to become a safe and knowledgeable practitioner of electrology.

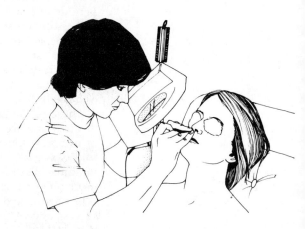

CLOSE UP OF FACIAL EPILATION

THE CLIENT

Before embarking on practical training in the techniques and organization of electrology, consideration should be given by the student to the nature of the work itself and the individuals who will seek the electrologist's skill. Just as in any other service profession, there has to be a desire to provide help of a very specialized kind to those people needing treatment. The client seeking relief from her hair problem may be distressed, depressed, or simply inconvenienced by her superfluous or unwanted hair. In severe cases, the disfigurement may have caused actual mental distress necessitating medical help. The problem may not be an isolated one, but associated with, or present as, a direct result of a physical change, illness or drug medication.

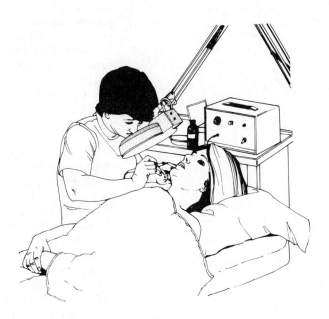

FACIAL EPILATION IN PROGRESS

Often the problem is simply linked to hormonal changes in the body, but that does not necessarily lessen the client's anxiety. Although the majority of clients will have only a cosmetic hair problem (that is, a problem of no medical interest), this does not relieve their embarrassment or make it any easier for them to come to terms with the condition. The electrologist must, therefore, be aware of the client's attitude towards the hair problem and seek to provide a solution as swiftly and skilfully as possible, with as little disruption to the client's normal life and appearance as possible.

One of the first difficulties to be experienced is persuading a client with a severe hair growth problem to allow the offending hairs to grow and become visible so that they can be treated. This may prove a real hurdle to progress if the client is intent on concealing the problem at all costs and resorts to temporary methods of hair removal which never permit the hairs to grow sufficiently to be dealt with permanently. A compromise between retaining the client's 'hair-free' appearance and having hairs visible enough for treatment has to be reached, and this relies greatly on the operator's skill in handling the client. Apart from slowing the progress of the hair removal, interference with the hair growth between treatments may alter the skin healing process and disrupt the overall programme by necessitating lengthy pauses between treatments to allow for skin recovery. Therefore, knowing the client and developing a method of client handling which ensures good co-operation in all aspects of the treatment, is as important as the technique itself. In fact, it *is* a part of the technique and has to be learnt as such.

Clients will come from every walk of life and the electrologist must be able to adapt to differing personalities and attitudes. Clients' feelings about their hair problems can vary from annoyance, to distress and embarrassment, or to severe anxiety and feelings of persecution that they should have been singled out in this way. The electrologist must, therefore, develop a calm and mature outlook towards her clients and their problems to avoid the work becoming emotionally wearing. Most clients, however, see the electrologist as the answer to their problems and adopt a positive attitude to resolving their unwanted hair growth situation. They place themselves in her hands and have faith in her abilities. The practitioner can foster this positive attitude with personal encouragement and a firm but sympathetic approach when progress is slow. For in its present form epilation is a *slow* treatment, but as yet it provides the only really permanent answer.

The electrologist can best help her clients by becoming as expert as possible, so that each session of treatment is as effective as it can possibly be and the clients can see a visible improvement. It is not only the *speed* of hair removal that needs to be considered here, however, but also the *accuracy* of probing and techniques generally, so that the effect of each application is maximized and hairs need only the minimum number of applications for complete destruction of the hair growth.

The main concern of the client is to be free of the hair problem and to achieve this without inconvenience, undue delay or embarrassment caused by her appearance while the treatment is in progress. If this can be achieved, the operator has justified the client's confidence in her professional abilities, and she can be proud of her work.

The clients who will become the life work of the electrologist have a real need for help and require handling with tact and understanding to obtain a permanent solution to their hair growth problems. Thus, a remedial influence underlies all aspects of electrology, and it can be thought of as work of a clinical nature.

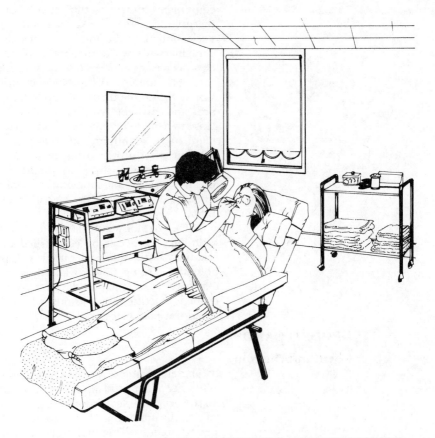

GENERAL CLINIC VIEW WORKING POSITION

THE WORKING ENVIRONMENT

The task of permanent hair removal is performed in a clinical setting, either in an independent practice or within a beauty therapy business. It may be carried out in association with a medical practice, or be a service offered in a large store alongside hairdressing and beauty facilities. Whatever the situation, the work in essence is always the same, though the bias towards cosmetic or remedial work may differ, according to the area of work which holds the most interest for the operator personally and which she wishes to develop.

The electrologist should provide a pleasant, light environment for treatment, one that will put the client at ease. A comfortable chair/couch, a trolley, an adjustable stool, illuminated magnification and the epilation equipment itself are all the components required for success. The epilation equipment comprises the actual short wave diathermy unit, normally known as the *epilation unit*, a selection of needle holders and needles, tweezers, containers for waste materials, lotions and powders, as well as a means of cleansing and sterilizing the tools required. All the small equipment can be stored within the treatment trolley, making a very neat and efficient working unit with everything close to hand. This ensures that preparation time is kept to a minimum, allowing the maximum amount of treatment time to be devoted to the actual application; this is an important point, with normal appointments being of only 15 to 20 minutes duration and the cost of treatment being high.

The electrology cubicle requires comparatively little space and can be established quickly with relatively little financial outlay compared to its potential earning power. The most essential and expensive component of the electrology unit is the trained practitioner, without whom the service could not take place.

RECORD CARDS

Client Information

The electrologist works on an individual basis with her clients, planning their treatment from start to finish—devising the best method of treatment, the duration of the applications, and the periods required between appointments to allow satisfactory healing to take place. It is responsible work and, in order to ensure good results, it is important for the operator to have adequate information about her clients so that she can make the correct treatment plan. Each client's treatment record and personal details should be listed on a **client's record card**, which provides a full account of progress and any special problems encountered. Most of the facts required will be supplied by the client at the initial consultation and will help the electrologist to diagnose the cause of the problem and its likely future development. This determines the form the treatment will take, gives an indication of the pattern of improvement that can be expected and provides guidance as to how long the treatment will take to resolve the condition satisfactorily.

NAME Mrs A. Jennings   ADDRESS 130 Brennan Road
Norton

DOCTOR Brinkwell   TEL. HOME 32416   WORK 32-72-81
Caldwell Practice

AGE & MEDICAL HISTORY 48
Hysterectomy at 41

CURRENT MEDICATIONS & TREATMENT None. No medical reason for
problem. Approval given for treatment.

PREVIOUS EPILATION No   SKIN CONDITION rather sensitive
& METHOD OF REMOVAL Chemical   due to use of chemical depilatories
depilatories - occasional waxing   and plucking
- plucking   HAIR CONDITION Dense, strong
growth affecting the chin and lip.

DATE	TREATMENT & COMMENTS	DATE	TREATMENT & COMMENTS
2.2.82	Consultation/10 min. Tr. Intensity 2-3	14.4.83	20 mins. Original and regrowth
16.2.82	20 min. Treatment. Intensity 2-3½		hairs treated. Intensity 1-3
31.2.82	20 min. Lip/Chin. No reactions		
13.3.82	20 min. Previously plucked hairs present		
27.3.82	20 min. Continuous clearance of original growth. Skin condition settled. Progress good.		

CLIENT'S RECORD CARD

Full consultation techniques (see Chapter 4) are not necessary at the initial stage of training, but the relevance of the information obtained to the successful outcome of the treatment must be understood right at the start. Judgement of the hair condition—whether medical referral is desirable or whether the problem falls within a 'normal' category—rests on this information. Therefore, skill in handling clients and obtaining information tactfully is as important as practical abilities. The interpretation of this client information slowly becomes established by studying the causes of superfluous hair growth and considering their relationship to the endocrine system (see Chapter 5). Initially, it is valuable to concentrate on normal hair growth patterns and to see how these alter in life. Then a deviation from the norm can be recognized more easily, and its pattern of behaviour assessed. Superfluous hairs can grow 'out of character' for their location and do not always follow a normal growth cycle. Superfluous hairs are often, in fact, not 'normal' hairs, but ones that have changed their strength, colour and shape in the follicle, a point which will be evident on the initial examination and should be recorded on the client's card. So, a major point in the first stage of hair diagnosis is to consider what is normal and understand how these hairs are structured and grow in the skin. Then, a comparison can be formed between normality and abnormality, and the correct plan of treatment can be worked out.

The details required initially include the client's name and initials (in case of duplication of the surname), address, telephone numbers—both at home and work—, the doctor's name and address and a brief medical history. Details of the hair and skin condition as first seen should also be recorded. Other points to note will be evidence of previous treatment, scarring, discoloration of the skin, any infection present, distorted hair growth and the presence of regrowth hairs. Certain information will have to be obtained from the client such as reactions to any previous treatment, skin healing abilities, the rate of the hair growth, etc. If the hairs have been removed just prior to the consultation by temporary methods (depilatory creams, plucking, etc.), the true extent of the superfluous hair problem can only be assessed from client information. It is important to remember, however, that this is a very inaccurate guide, and this should be explained fully to the client at the initial examination (see Chapter 4). For, if the hairs are normally plucked as they emerge from the skin, both the client and the operator may well be surprised as to the true extent of the problem. Hairs can take up to six weeks to grow back up the follicle after plucking, and, therefore, new hairs will *appear* to emerge during the epilation treatment, possibly causing the client to think of them as 'new' hairs, whereas they are, in fact, hairs that would have been present initially had they not been removed by temporary interference with the hair growth.

This is one reason why it is not possible to give the client an *accurate* idea of the length of time it will take to resolve her hair problem. The picture presented in early treatment sessions often proves to be totally inaccurate as the weeks progress and the hairs are permitted to grow. It will be seen later (see Chapter 2) how this can be achieved without embarrassment to the client.

The operator's assessment of her client's hair condition and its subsequent treatment is based largely on experience. It is always wise to err on the side of caution as to the skin's tolerance to diathermy (heat) epilation treatment, bearing in mind that it is *the skin*, and *its sensitivity*, that determine the current intensity that can be used in the process of hair destruction.

Treatment Details

Treatment details are recorded after the initial appointment to act as a guide to subsequent sessions. Every appointment is recorded in detail, as well as any special points of relevance to future applications. The current intensity used, the epilation unit used (if a choice is available), the spacing of the probes and the area treated are all recorded. This last point is very important in order to avoid treating the same area twice before the underlying tissues have healed. It may not be possible to tell which areas have already been treated simply by looking at the skin, and the addition of further epilation work, prematurely, could cause dehydration resulting in pitting and scarring. This lack of attention to treatment spacing is a major cause of scarring, brought about by both the client's anxiety to be rid of her problem and by the electrologist's wish to help her towards a solution. Unfortunately, overdoing treatment, by placing the probes too close together or giving treatment sessions too frequently, only causes poor results and skin damage. Often, if over-treatment has occurred, recovery periods have to be inserted into the treatment plan programme to permit the skin to heal correctly. This slows the progress of the entire plan and can be very depressing for the client, and should, therefore be avoided if at all possible. The electrologist should remember that a good result overall is needed, not necessarily the fastest result if that means skin damage is going to occur. As a professional electrologist, the operator should be in complete control of the treatment timing and, using the client's card as a reference, should space the applications and their durations as *she* sees best.

A complete picture of the client is thus built up from her client's record card—her personal details, any problems of treatment which might make adjustments necessary and a complete record of the epilation received (dates, durations, results). If the client's medical background has an obvious bearing on her hair condition, it may be necessary to obtain further details from her doctor (see Chapter 5).

ANATOMY OF THE HAIR FOLLICLE

In order to accomplish the ideal combination of maximum destruction of the hair follicle with minimum skin damage, it is important to understand the physiology of the hair-producing *follicle*. The histology or anatomy of the follicle is best understood by considering a fully active follicle, that is one in the most extended stage of the growth cycle. This stage, known as *anagen*, is the active growth stage which lasts for the majority of the hair's life cycle before it degenerates and falls out.

The follicle and the hair have to be considered as one unit, often referred to as the *philo-sebaceous unit*, indicating the follicle's dual role of hair production and skin lubrication. The follicle produces the hair according to messages received via its blood supply, and discards it eventually through shedding. It then rests prior to forming a replacement hair. This process of growth, rest and replacement, known as the *hair growth cycle*, will be considered briefly at this stage to permit the description of practical techniques, but it will be studied in detail in Chapter 3.

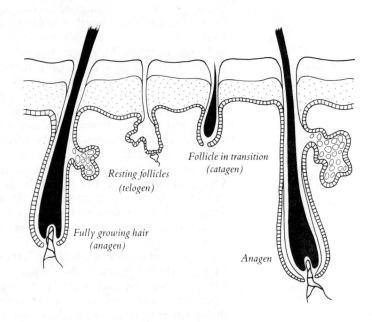

Resting follicles
(telogen)

Follicle in transition
(catagen)

Fully growing hair
(anagen)

Anagen

SIMPLE HAIR GROWTH CYCLE

It is possible to think of a hair follicle as a pocket in the skin, as if a finger had been pushed down into the deeper layers of the skin to provide a cavity from which the hair could grow. The hair follicle throughout its depth is lined with cells of the *epidermis*, the skin's surface layer, which at the lower bulb end of the follicle become the *tissue sheath*, surrounding the hair and being firmly bonded to it.

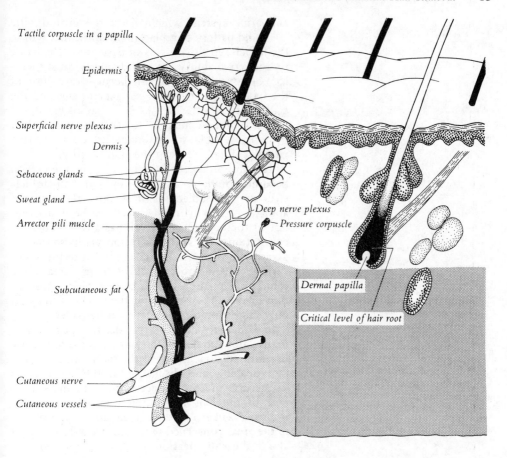

Tactile corpuscle in a papilla

Epidermis

Superficial nerve plexus

Dermis

Sebaceous glands

Sweat gland

Arrector pili muscle

Subcutaneous fat

Cutaneous nerve

Cutaneous vessels

Deep nerve plexus

Pressure corpuscle

Dermal papilla

Critical level of hair root

SECTION OF A HAIR IN A FOLLICLE

If a normal hair follicle structure is bisected longitudinally, the various areas can be clearly seen. The hair itself grows from an area of cells at the base of the follicle known as the *matrix* area. The activity centre of the matrix region is known as the *dermal papilla*, a concave shaped area of intense cellular activity inside the bulb of the forming hair. Both the epidermis and the dermal papilla are affected by the epilation process and so are of importance.

The dermal papilla and indeed the whole matrix area is well supplied with small blood vessels and nerve endings. The blood supply is usually represented diagrammatically as a capillary loop, although it is in fact made up of many tiny blood vessels intermeshed around the follicle. This *vascularity* is vital to the well-being of the hair follicle and the hair structure, providing the means of nutrition necessary to sustain or grow a hair, and acts as the carrier of hormonal messages from the endocrine system which direct the growth, life cycle and pattern of replacement of the hair within the follicle. In the process of destroying the hair's reproductive ability, its blood supply must therefore be cut off. After the diathermy destruction of the hair bulb and matrix has taken place and the cauterization of the blood vessels has occurred, the follicle, though unable to sustain future hair growth, is able to maintain its own reduced vascular supply to keep the skin healthy.

The importance of accuracy in hair epilation becomes obvious as the skin and hair follicle structure is studied, as it is only the follicle's ability to grow hairs that needs to be destroyed, not its total existence. It still has a role to play in connection with skin lubrication via its sebaceous glands and their output of sebum on to the skin's surface. The destruction of the matrix area of the follicle by epilation should be seen as an intervention or disruption of *part* of the follicle's function only, and should not affect its other roles.

In order to destroy the dermal papilla and matrix area and detach the hair from the follicle by breaking its attachment to the tissue sheath, accurate probing and discharge of the short wave diathermy current are necessary. If the moist bulb area of the hair is accurately probed, its very moisture will attract the current and concentrate it in the areas concerned with hair growth, bringing about the cauterization of those areas and also reducing unwanted current seepage. The entire

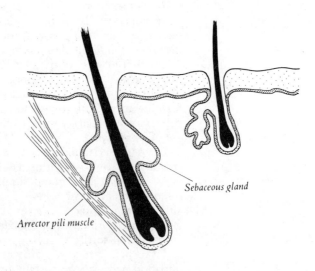

COMPARISON OF NORMAL AND REGROWTH HAIR

matrix area of the hair follicle, surrounding and beneath the hair bulb, has to be cauterized by the heat reaction and made ineffective. If the hair growth is very strong, it may well not be possible to use the necessary amount of diathermy current to accomplish total destruction without undue skin damage, skin burns, etc. In this instance, although the cauterized hair may be removed and lifted from the follicle freely, the matrix and dermal papilla areas may revive and still have the necessary resources to grow another hair. This hair will be finer in texture, paler in colour and may also be slightly distorted due to the damaged nature of the follicle. This *regrowth hair* is always recognizable and needs very little further treatment to accomplish complete removal.

It is possible to study the various components of the philo-sebaceous structure and to observe where they lie in relation to one another by considering the hair follicle in a diagrammatic form. However, it does not provide a complete picture of how the hair follicles are placed within the skin or show their diversity of angles and depths. For this, it is necessary to study a slide of a cross-section of the skin and hairs which shows clearly the indentations of the surface layers, called the *papillary processes*, and how the follicles relate to these depressions in the skin's surface. Such an example of the hairs' positions show far more

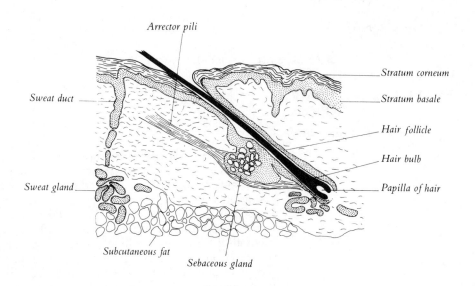

HAIR IN ANAGEN

accurately why careful probing of the follicle is necessary and why the operator requires a good sense of touch to guide the probe into the correct area at the base of the hair. It also explains why many hairs are not accurately probed, and hence, not being destroyed, regrow again after treatment.

It is also important, when considering normal hairs *in situ* (in the skin), to realize that the hair follicles will differ in structure, depending on the hair type—whether curly, frizzy, negroid, etc. Racial differences will contribute to this variety of hair structures and follicles. Excessively curly or negroid hair has curved or distorted follicles which are almost impossible to probe with traditional needle-probe methods and are, therefore, very difficult to treat.

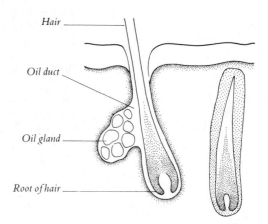

Mongoloid scalp hair

Negroid scalp hair

Vertical section of the scalp

HAIR ANGLES AND PAPILLARY PROCESSES

EVALUATION OF HAIR GROWTH

Correct Terminology

It has been seen that hairs differ according to genetic factors, racial tendencies, etc., and that it is important to evaluate or assess the hair growth condition for clinic record purposes in order to devise a treatment plan. Hairs also differ in terms of their location on the body, and this affects the method of treatment, probing angles, positioning of the client and so on. In order to be able to record accurately the hair condition it is necessary to understand and use the correct terminology in relation to the hair growth.

Superfluous hair growth is a general term used to describe any unwanted hair condition.

Lanugo hair is that formed on the foetus (unborn child) while in the womb. This fine primary hair, which lacks a *medulla*, is mainly shed shortly after birth, to be replaced by the permanent hair. Hair that is being lost through baldness on the scalp can be seen to revert to *lanugo-type* primary hair prior to its final disappearance.

Vellus hair growth is fine and soft and covers most areas of the body except the palms of the hands, soles of the feet, the lips and the genital areas. There is confusion between the terms *vellus* and *lanugo* hair, with either of them being used (incorrectly) to describe any fine downy hair growth.

Terminal hairs are coarse visible hairs found on the scalp, axilla (armpits) and pubic areas. Long coarse hairs which grow out of character for their location may be classed terminal hairs, for example, strong hairs around the female nipples.

Sexual hairs are *terminal-type hairs* which grow as a result of hormonal changes at puberty. In males, this growth includes hair in the armpits, pubic hair and beard and chest hair. In females, normal sexual development includes the growth of armpit and pubic hair.

Club hairs are those which appear to have a club-like formation when removed by epilation or when shed naturally from the follicle. The hair bulb has disintegrated, lost its bulb-like root, become fragmented and rounded, club-like in form.

Regrowth hairs are those which grow after epilation has taken place and partial destruction of the follicles has occurred. These hairs are finer then the original hairs, and are also paler in colour and shallowly placed in the skin.

Ingrowing hairs are those which, on emerging from the mouth of the hair follicle, either grow along under the skin's surface or turn back into the follicle opening and become compacted. These hairs can cause irritation or become infected. They are often a result of waxing or plucking, or caused by some other distortion of the follicle. The epilation process can occasionally cause them to occur when the regrowth hair emerges.

The Hair Growth Cycle

In later chapters, it will be necessary to consider how the hair is formed and the factors which govern its growth and behaviour in life. A careful appraisal of its renewal process will also be necessary, but initially a simple understanding of the growth cycle will enable the practical techniques to progress.

The growth pattern of the hair can be studied starting from any stage in the cycle, as in normal health it is a continuous process of loss and replacement. The hairs in any area will be found to be in a variety of stages in the growth cycle, as can be clearly seen if they are removed forcibly by plucking or waxing (mass plucking). Some hairs will be seen to have long root structures with milky looking tissue sheaths surrounding them, while others will have shallow club-like roots without tissue sheaths. There will be a vast discrepancy in the overall form and depth of the hairs since each hair follicle obeys its own growth cycle and replacement pattern. For instance, coarse terminal hairs on the head have a different replacement rate from the fine vellus hairs on the body, or from those which have a special task to perform, such as the eye lashes or brows. Each individual hair follows a pattern dictated by internal messages received via the blood stream from the endocrine system of the body. These hormonal messages dictate the growth, rest and renewal cycles of the hair follicle, and these are represented by three stages in the growth cycle:

Growing hair follicles are said to be in **anagen**.

The transitionary or changing phase is known as **catagen**.

Resting hair follicles are said to be in **telogen**.

The **anagen stage** is the most active, during which the follicle elongates to six times its original depth and forms a new, strong hair growth, which may remain intact for months or years depending on its location and function.

When hormonal influences indicate that replacement is necessary, the anagen hair is shed and the follicle enters a period of change and adjustment known as **catagen**, which is seen as a transitionary phase between 'growth and activity' and 'rest'.

The follicle, now a simpler, more shallow structure, remains in a state of rest and inactivity, and this period of quiescence and recuperation, known as **telogen**, continues until such time as that follicle is once more prompted into activity to regenerate a new hair.

This orderly and complex process ensures that replacement hairs are present when required, and regrowth should equal normal loss from shedding in the healthy individual. Hereditary and genetic factors do, of course, influence hair growth pat-

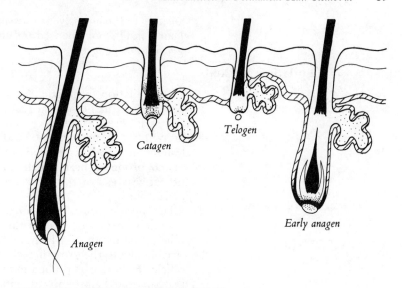

Catagen

Telogen

Early anagen

Anagen

DIFFERENT STAGES OF HAIR GROWTH

terns as can be seen in the pattern of male baldness, where the overall hair growth of an individual is dictated by background factors over which there is no personal control. But it is very evident that growth patterns, both in normal health and in illness or physical abnormality, are directly influenced by the **endocrine system**, and the electrologist should be aware of this relationship between hair growth and physical health. Although it will not be her responsibility to diagnose hair irregularities associated with illness, it is important for her to be aware that a link does exist.

METHODS OF HAIR DESTRUCTION

Several factors have to be present for unwanted hairs to be successfully and permanently removed without skin damage. Firstly, it is necessary to generate sufficient destructive power around the dermal papilla to render the follicle incapable of producing another hair. Secondly, and of equal importance if the skin is to remain undamaged in the destructive process, this force must be accurately positioned so that adjacent tissues do not suffer undue damage. Some skin damage to the tissues directly associated with, or positioned around, the matrix area is inevitable, but this should not affect the skin's surface appearance. In addition, the treatment should be performed as quickly and painlessly as possible, so that the client is not inconvenienced and soon feels encouraged by her progress.

Epilation Method

The epilation technique uses a high frequency, short wave diathermy current which produces heat as its destructive force. This current, when directed via a fine, metal needle probe to the desired area and discharged for a fraction of a second produces heat which, in turn, cauterizes the active areas of the follicle and renders them ineffective.

The needle must, therefore, be placed very accurately in order to reach the base of the hair follicle, the depth of which, as has been seen, is variable due to the growth cycle of the hair in the follicle. Each hair is probed individually, and the treated, dead hair removed with forceps (finely balanced tweezers). Thus, it can be seen that epilation is a slow method with no instant results, but one which can eventually offer a permanent solution to the problem.

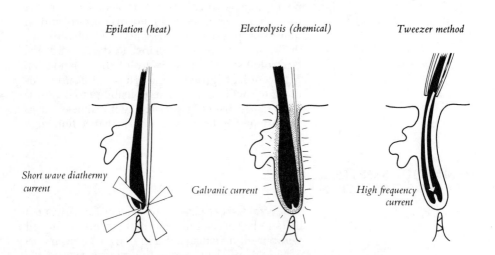

Epilation (heat)   *Electrolysis (chemical)*   *Tweezer method*

Short wave diathermy current   *Galvanic current*   *High frequency current*

METHODS OF HAIR DESTRUCTION

Electrolysis Method

This method of treatment uses a direct galvanic current introduced via the negative pole, to bring about chemical destruction of the active part of the follicle. Tissue destruction occurs as a result of the caustic action of sodium hydroxide formed at the needle point as a reaction to the skin tissues. The destruction occurs slowly—taking from a few seconds to several minutes to produce the effect needed—and the decomposition allows the treated hair to be removed without resistance. This lack of resistance indicates that the hair has lost its mechanical attachment to the follicle and that destruction of the active, germinative portion of the follicle has occurred.

Electrolysis is a slower process than epilation and has been largely superseded by it, but it has advantages in certain instances. Distorted follicles, or those of abnormal activity, may benefit from treatment by electrolysis. In cases where electrical currents may not be used, that is where epilation is contra-indicated (not considered suitable), the chemical method offers a useful alternative. For instance, clients who have certain illnesses, such as epilepsy, or are of a nervous disposition, or have a hair growth condition involving distortion of the hair follicles, may all use the electrolysis (galvanic) method of removal to advantage. It is also often used for individual problem hairs within a treatment plan based on the faster epilation method.

Tweezer Method

Although the tweezer method of hair removal is still very widely used, it is not currently considered by the electrology profession to give the proven results necessary to class it as a method of *permanent* hair removal. This controversial technique, however, is promoted as such, and commonly believed to be capable of giving the desired results quickly and without discomfort. That this is often *not* the case may reflect badly on the electrology profession and could lead to a loss of confidence by the general public. For this reason, electrologists have up to now been very critical of this method of treatment, and especially of the form of promotion which claims it to be an unskilled task, leaving the client to the mercies of untrained operators.

Electrologists should acquaint themselves with this method of hair removal and evaluate its advantages and disadvantages. Then, if it is found not to provide a permanent method of hair destruction, it should have no place in professional electrology and should be rejected.

The tweezer method utilizes a high frequency current to effect the hair destruction, using the hair as the route to the hair root and dermal papilla. In principle, the technique of tweezer epilation has many advantages and seeks both to reduce the pain element and minimize the area affected by the application. Unfortunately, because the hair is a very poor conductor the current is easily diverted from its path to the hair bulb, and the destructive effect on the dermal papilla is reduced. The moisture of the hair bulb is thought to attract the current, but results would seem to show that a large percentage of the current is lost on the skin's surface, deflected through surface moisture, or blocked by natural oils, and *permanent* results have not yet been achieved.

The process of tweezer hair removal is different in principle from the so-called traditional or needle methods, and, with additional research, it is possible that it can be improved to become not only safe, but also effective.

Thus it can be seen from this brief comparison of the methods available that at present needle probing offers the best results and the epilation method is the most effective and the most widely used in professional electrology. Therefore, apart from providing a theoretical consideration of the electrolysis and tweezer methods, this book will concentrate on epilation, and all techniques and principles of hair removal practice will refer exclusively to epilation unless otherwise stated.

Future Methods of Hair Removal

At present virtually all permanent hair removal is accomplished by the electrical heat method (epilation). However, this will undoubtedly change and electrologists should be alert to new developments that can be tested by clinical trials.

Laser beams are currently being considered as a tool for permanent hair removal, having already been used experimentally in the removal of livid birth marks (port wine stains) with considerable success. However, the problem of controlling the force—that is, how to get sufficient power to the area to achieve the destruction while limiting its damaging effects on surrounding skin tissues—would seem to be a major obstacle.

EQUIPMENT

In order to understand the effects of a short wave diathermy unit used for epilation purposes, it is best first to consider it in its simplest form. Diathermy (heat) is used in medicine for many purposes, and the destructive burning effect is only one of its many applications. The equipment provides a destructive, cauterizing force which coagulates the tissues in a controlled manner if applied accurately by means of a probe (needle). It is used medically for cauterizing wounds, sealing small blood vessels during surgery and removing warts, moles, etc.—all with the assistance of an anaesthetic. Since the electrologist is not permitted to use local anaesthetics in her work, accuracy is obviously essential to minimize the client's discomfort during treatment. If epilation is carried out in a hospital, however, under direct medical supervision, then the electrologist may have the benefit of working with local anaesthetics, administered by medical staff.

Therefore, diathermy, though so useful in its results, is a *destructive force with painful effects* and must be applied with care and due regard for the client's feelings.

The equipment available for epilation is very varied, but it always contains a short wave diathermy unit—the basic element necessary for hair destruction. It is possible to consider this unit as essentially a **power source**, with a means of controlling the amount of current used (the **intensity control**), and a means of applying the current to the tissues accurately (a **needle holder with needle**). There are two methods of controlling the current in common use: (1) by means of a **finger button** on the needle holder and (2) by a **foot-switch** connection. Personal preference will decide the best method for the individual operator, but it is important to be proficient in both methods to permit flexibility of employment. In different parts of the world, one system or the other dominates, and most of the equipment produced locally will follow this preference, being either entirely foot-switch (as in the USA) or finger button (as in the UK). Therefore, in

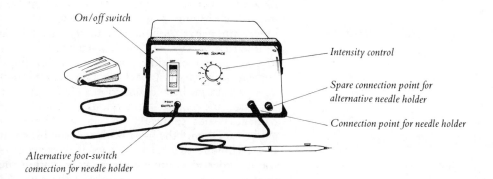

On/off switch

Intensity control

Spare connection point for alternative needle holder

Connection point for needle holder

Alternative foot-switch connection for needle holder

SHORT WAVE DIATHERMY EPILATION UNIT

training it is useful to gain equal proficiency in both methods so that the transition from one to the other can be made easily.

Points to look for in an epilation unit on which your livelihood will depend are:

reliability

sturdy construction

simplicity of design (the fewer parts to go wrong, the less likely is malfunction or intermittent performance)

safety features (to guard against using too much current, and to prevent the current flowing when not required)

low pain element for clients

easy controls (well-positioned, easy to understand and use)

clinical appearance (neat size, modern design, easy to clean)

firm connections (easy-to-handle small equipment, needle holders, foot-switch connection, etc.)

The equipment's capacity to perform hair destruction quickly and with minimum discomfort relies to a large extent on the operator's skill in practical techniques. However, different epilation units, using slightly different levels of high frequency current, can alter the sensation experienced by the client. Modern advances in equipment have concentrated on this pain-reducing aspect and have succeeded in making it possible to achieve hair destruction very quickly with a high-powered unit, applying a white hot cautery for a fraction of a second and producing very little pain or skin reaction. Operators very skilled in probing, controlling the current discharge and handling the skin, can work with these units without causing skin damage, while producing excellent results. Initially, however, it is wise to use a lower, slower form of epilation technique, with a basic epilation unit which produces the same result in a slightly longer time, but without risk to the client. The simple rule of *low and slow* (low current, slow or longer application time) or *high and fast* (high current strength, fast or brief application time) both result in hair destruction. However, the high-fast rule requires tremendous accuracy if skin damage is not to result, and it should not be applied at all until the basic skills are established. It is a technique that all professional electrologists use in order to complete more work within the treatment period, while minimizing the pain element and skin reaction. It is a technique to aspire to as practical skill and knowledge increase.

Chapter 2

Practical Training in Epilation Techniques

THE WORKING POSITION

The ideal working position is one that allows the operator to work in a relaxed manner and to give her full attention to the client without distractions. She must, therefore, be comfortable, not under strain, able to see clearly the area under treatment and have all the equipment within easy reach. This attention to comfort and accessibility enables the operator to concentrate fully on the epilation task itself, and improves her probing skill and working speed, thus maximizing the effects of the application and allowing each probe to be really effective.

Once the operator is familiar with her own ideal working position and is practised in setting it up quickly, she will then be able to duplicate it whenever necessary and to adapt facilities to suit her own style of operating. This will be most helpful when working in different clinic situations or hospital wards, or when offering electrology on a mobile basis within the clients' homes.

The couch, trolley, magnifier, basic epilation unit and stool are the operator's working tools, and together with the small equipment, commodities, etc., form the epilation **working unit or position**.

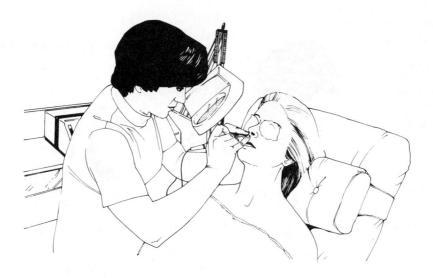

WORKING POSITION: FACIAL

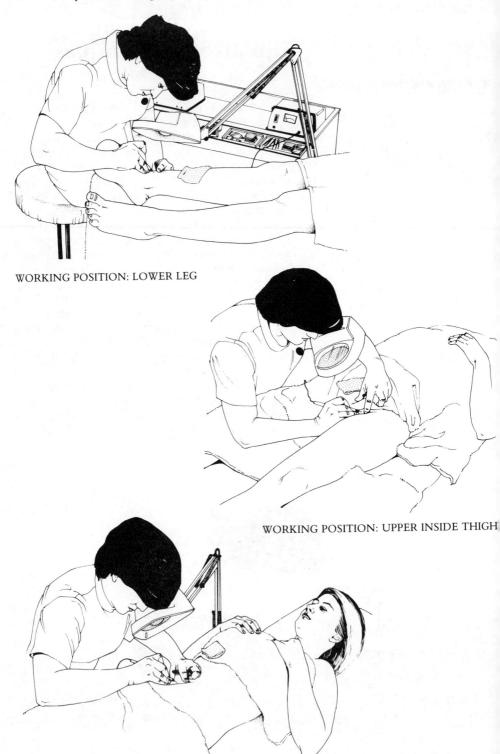

WORKING POSITION: LOWER LEG

WORKING POSITION: UPPER INSIDE THIGH

WORKING POSITION: ABDOMEN

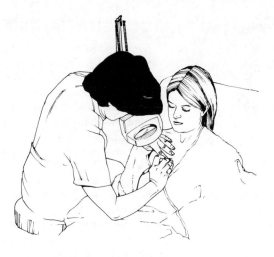

WORKING POSITION: BREAST

The Epilation Couch

An adjustable couch which permits correct positioning of the client for electrology is a valuable aid and well worth the initial expense. It allows extended periods of treatment (such as in leg epilation) to be undertaken without strain on the client or the operator and, in conjunction with a revolving stool, permits all areas of the client to be treated comfortably. It avoids operator fatigue caused by back strain resulting from poor positioning and ensures that a satisfactory level of work is maintained. If the operator is not comfortable, then her work will not be her best and the client will suffer.

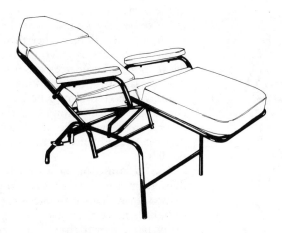

THE EPILATION COUCH

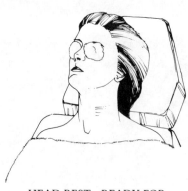

HEAD REST—READY FOR
THROAT EPILATION

Important points to consider when purchasing a couch are:

(1) the shape of the head rest to allow easy access to the client's lip and chin areas without straining or leaning on the client;
(2) ability to position the head rest accurately and fix it at different angles to permit free access to the throat and under-jaw areas;
(3) a height adjustment to allow the operator to treat legs without stooping;
(4) the overall comfort and padding of the couch to increase the relaxation of the client, thus helping to reduce general anxiety concerning the treatment.

The operator will spend such a lot of her working life at the couch side that it is well worth taking time and money to find the ideal couch/chair to suit her own requirements.

The Illuminated Magnifier

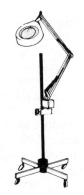

FLOOR-STANDING MAGNIFIER

The illuminated magnifier provides a source of constant light for the operator and acts as a breath shield between her and her client. Natural daylight, if constant, is ideal as it gives the clearest vision without distortion or glare. The illuminated magnifier, however, is a good substitute, and it also magnifies fine hairs, such as those found on the upper lip, enabling the operator to work accurately for longer periods without eyestrain. Magnifiers come in various models—floor-standing, trolley-mounted, part of an equipment system arrangement, or wall-mounted. The wall-mounted version, though space saving, makes it necessary to completely reposition the client and couch whenever body work has to be done which, in the confines of a small treatment cubicle, could prove to be very inconvenient. The client has to be brought to the light, rather than the light to the client, in this instance. Where the work is mainly facial, fixed illuminators are not a disadvantage, but can save precious working space. Within the training situation also, where open-plan training clinics are usually found, wall-mounted magnifiers are very useful and seem to suffer less damage in daily use than do the floor-standing models.

The illumination is normally provided by a fluorescent tube, either in a strip or horseshoe-shaped form. This provides a shadow-free source of light beneath the magnifying glass surface, and really aids the operator in her work. Even electrologists with excellent eyesight should get into the

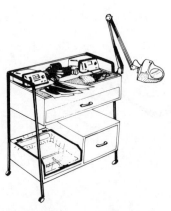

TROLLEY-MOUNTED MAGNIFIER

habit of working with a magnifier. It might seem awkward at first, but it soon becomes part of the routine and does save eyestrain.

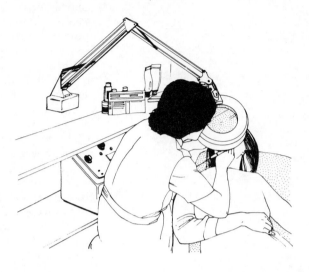

WALL-MOUNTED MAGNIFIER

The Epilation Unit

As has been seen, the basic components of any epilation unit are very similar. Choice of machine will depend on personal taste and availability of units, plus, of course, cost. Before they can be sold, machines have to meet the manufacturing and safety standards laid down by the bureau of standards in the country of origin. This does not necessarily mean that they will meet the safety standards set by another country, however, and so this point must be checked with the health authorities where the practice is planned.

In the USA, the Food and Drug Administration, through their Medical Devices Section, indicates which epilation units are satisfactory for use by the qualified electrologist. In other parts of the world, the UK, South Africa, Australia, Canada, for instance, the professional electrology associations work in liaison with health and medical and dental councils to give advice and guidance to their members regarding satisfactory and safe units. Most established manufacturers of epilation equipment work closely with the authorities to provide apparatus that not only fits the industry's requirements, but also satisfies the legal requirements for safeguarding the clients' welfare.

CONTROLS ON THE EPILATION
EQUIPMENT

It is essential to understand what each of the controls on an epilation machine is for, and to become familiar with their use. This helps to avoid confusion later on when sophisticated units are used, and improves the efficiency of the work.

When using a destructive force such as diathermy without medical qualifications, it is imperative that errors be avoided if public confidence in the service is to be maintained. With that point in mind, many manufacturers have built into their machines additional safety features to guard against operator error or electrical malfunction.

The controls comprise an **intensity control, connection sockets for the needle holder and foot-switch** (if applicable), a **pilot light**, an **on/off switch** and a **display panel** or **meter** to indicate the actual amount of current flowing. Some models may also include a **pre-set timing control**, which provides a means of automatically cutting off the current flow after a predetermined period of time.

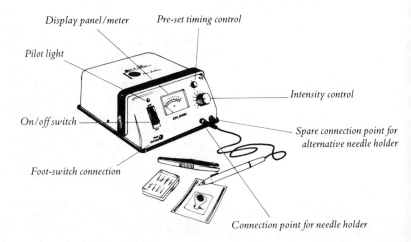

Display panel/meter   Pre-set timing control

Pilot light

Intensity control

On/off switch

Spare connection point for
alternative needle holder

Foot-switch connection

Connection point for needle holder

EPILATION MACHINE

The epilation unit should be positioned close to the operator on a trolley placed on the working side of the client. This avoids the machine's connecting flexes trailing across the client during treatment, and allows the operator to make minute current intensity adjustments whenever necessary during the application. This adjustment of the controls becomes almost an extension of the probing sequence, and they must, therefore, be close to hand to avoid the operator having to reposition herself during the application.

Intensity Control

The intensity control may be graduated in a number of different ways, normally 1 to 10, or 10 to 100, and it should be thought of as a gauge to show the amount of current that will flow when the connection through to the needle holder is made. This information can be confirmed on a milliamp meter incorporated into some designs of epilation unit. If there are a number of models in use, the epilation model or type and the intensity levels used should be carefully recorded on the client's card, to avoid errors occurring, particularly if more than one operator may be involved in the client's treatment.

Needle Holder and Foot-switch Connections

Connections to the needle holder and foot-switch are normally by means of sockets from which the flexes may be detached for safety at the end of treatment sessions or when the unit has to be moved. If the machine has a foot-switch only, this connection may well be built into the unit, and be permanently connected, with only the needle holder detachable.

Pilot Light

The pilot light indicates when the unit has power flowing to it and gives valuable guidance as to the possible cause of malfunction or intermittent performance. It also prevents the unit being left switched on inadvertently between epilation sessions or overnight. On some epilation units the pilot light also plays a part in the testing of the power to the needle point, indicating that the flow sequence is correct and all the connection points are firm and allowing a good transmission of current through to the needle tip.

Timing Controls

Pre-set timing facilities are available on many machines, and can be useful in preventing over-treatment of individual hair follicles where a large number of very similar hairs are being treated, such as in leg hair treatment. Normally, however, the professional electrologist prefers to rely on her own judgement regarding the duration of the current application to the hair follicle, as the timing required to treat each individual hair can be so variable.

The Trolley

The trolley provides storage for all the small equipment and commodities needed in the epilation process and acts as a mobile base for the epilation machine, allowing it to be moved freely around the client. Ideally, the small equipment—needle holder, needles, forceps, spare needle holder, chucks, etc.—should be stored in a drawer compartment on the trolley for safety and hygiene, as they are easily broken and must be kept in a sterile condition. A closed container acts as a good substitute if a drawer is not available.

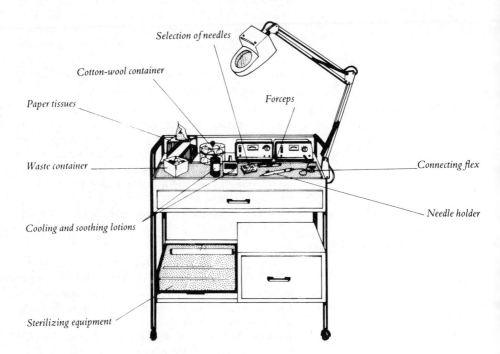

Selection of needles

Cotton-wool container

Paper tissues

Forceps

Waste container

Connecting flex

Needle holder

Cooling and soothing lotions

Sterilizing equipment

The Small Equipment

The small equipment includes a needle holder, connecting flex, a selection of needles for differing hair conditions, forceps for removing the hairs after destruction, sterilizing equipment, cotton-wool in a closed container, paper tissues, container for waste, as well as cooling and soothing lotions for skin preparation and aftercare.

THE NEEDLE HOLDER

The needle holder may be of a type either with or without a button connection, the latter being for use with a foot-switch to connect the power. The holder should be neat and easy to hold and should fit the operator's hand comfortably. It should be short in length so that it can reach areas not easily accessible, such as under the jaw bone, without touching or causing discomfort to the client, or causing any restriction in the actual probe of the follicle. Furthermore, a small needle holder makes it very much easier to work behind the confines of the magnifier without undue restriction of movement. The neater the movements of the epilation probing sequence, the faster will be the rate of removals and thus the more efficient the process.

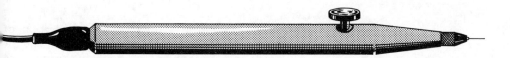

BUTTON-TYPE NEEDLE HOLDER

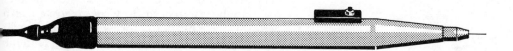

SWITCH-CONTROLLED NEEDLE HOLDER

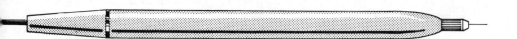

FOOT-SWITCH NEEDLE HOLDER

The needle holder is so important to a good technique that a cumbersome holder, if provided with the epilation machine, should be replaced with the correct tool for the job. This may entail altering the connecting portion of the flex to fit a different type of connection socket on the machine, but this is a small electrical task which is well worth having done in order to get a needle holder which feels right in the hand. Most electrologists like to keep their personal needle holder together with a pair of forceps, as part of their own small equipment, to use whenever and wherever they are working.

The complete needle holder has several parts: the connection, the flex, the holder with its top section or chuck, the cap, the needle and the protective cover. The top section of the holder, often referred to as the chuck, must be able to accept the chosen needle so that a firm connection is possible in order to avoid movement of the needle and loss of current at the connection. Some needle holders are able to take any needle, working on a screwhold principle to grasp the needle and hold it firm, but these holders, unfortunately, are rare.

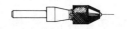

NEEDLE HOLDER CHUCK

THE NEEDLE

The equipment should contain a selection of needles of varying sizes and diameters suitable for work on different hair conditions. In common use are fine steel needles set into larger bases for stability—these needles are normally known as *Ferrie needles*. Platinum needles were also popular at one time, but are too fragile for training purposes and even in professional hands have a very short life. Longer, insulated steel needles (commonly referred to as *German needles*) also perform the epilation process extremely well, especially on delicate skin, but their extreme flexibility makes them more difficult to use, especially for a less experienced operator.

All fine needles in their correct needle holder will complete the epilation task satisfactorily and it is useful to have a range to choose from for the different hair and skin conditions that will present themselves. The main difference between needles is durability and, therefore, the Ferrie needle is the most common choice both in training and practice as it combines strength with flexibility and is available in a range of diameters to suit all hair conditions.

The length of the Ferrie needle remains constant, but it is available in a range of diameters or thicknesses shown as a scale from .003 to .006, with the .004 or .005 needles being the ones in most general use. Needles of the .003 diameter, being very fine and flexible, are used only for very difficult fine hair growth, while .006 needles, which are thicker and more rigid, are the ideal choice for strong hair growth such as is found on the legs, where high current intensities are used for longer sessions of treatment.

It has been noted that some needle holders are capable of taking any needle, but more commonly, the top connection piece of the holder must match the needle and be chosen specifically

Ferrie steel
.003 diameter

.004 diameter

.005 diameter

.006 diameter

Steel needle

Insulated needle—
rounded probe—
available in .003 to
.006 diameter

Insulated needle
(German), longer length,
only one diameter,
equivalent of .004

Platinum needle—
no base shank

SELECTION OF NEEDLES

Chuck   *Cap*

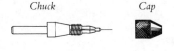

POSITIONING OF NEEDLE IN
CHUCK

EPILATION FORCEPS

for it. This means, for instance, that Ferrie and German insulated needles cannot be interchanged as they have different shanks or bases to the needles, and the claws of the needle holder cannot grasp them both equally well. However, it is possible to interchange additional chucks or top sections of the needle holders simply and quickly. The needle is then held by metal claws at the top of the chuck which can be tightened gently with a pair of ordinary tweezers or by finger pressure if the connection becomes loose from usage. It is essential that the contact is firm, as, apart from the risk of needle movement during the actual probe and discharge of current, a poor connection may well hinder the current from flowing correctly to the needle tip, thus preventing proper destruction of the hair.

Epilation forceps are finely balanced, surgical tweezers which are used to remove the dead epilated hair from the follicle. They are held in the operator's hand, normally balanced between the thumb and the index finger of the hand holding the skin, ready for use after epilation of each hair. The positioning of the forceps is an individual matter, but practice has shown that in training it is preferable to concentrate on working with the forceps in this position initially, to free other parts of the holding hand for stretching, rolling or steadying the skin while the probe is being made.

The epilation forceps should not be used for any purpose other than epilation, or the grip of the

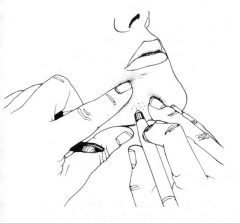

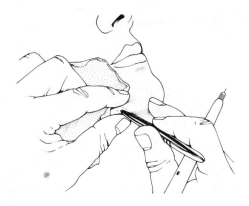

NEEDLE IN USE. FORCEPS IN OTHER HAND   FORCEPS IN USE

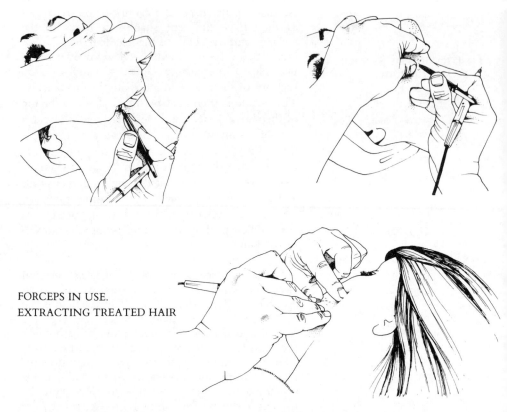

FORCEPS IN USE.
EXTRACTING TREATED HAIR

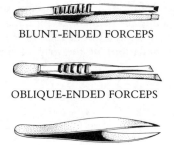

BLUNT-ENDED FORCEPS

OBLIQUE-ENDED FORCEPS

POINTED FORCEPS

points will be lost, thereby reducing the operator's speed. Forceps are available in pointed, oblique- and blunt-ended versions to suit different patterns and distribution of hair growth. The most popular are the oblique-ended forceps, because they can be used at different angles, both to pick out the hairs from intricate, densely packed growth, and for more general work.

Small precision forceps can be extremely hard to find and, once obtained, tend to be kept and treasured by the operator, recognized as one of the excellent tools that help to obtain good, fast results.

SETTING UP THE WORKING POSITION

Practice in setting up the working position increases familiarity with the equipment and allows the routine of work to become automatic. This then frees the operator to pay complete attention to the client and her problem and to concentrate fully on her practical techniques rather than being anxious about her positioning. It also enhances safety because, if safety checks become automatic at an early stage in training, they will not be forgotten in the pace of daily clinic practice, when the operator is under pressure to work fast, or is tired at the end of a long day.

Even though, in the early stages of training, the electrologist will not be using the actual diathermy current of the machine until probing skills are developed, it is advisable to practise setting up the entire epilation working unit. Then, at a later date, the current can be added into the sequence with minimum disruption to the techniques already acquired, without affecting the confidence that has been built up. This is an important point, as confident handling of the equipment is one of the first essentials to skill and accuracy in electrology. An electrologist who has never achieved control over her needle holder and forceps will never attain the levels of skill or speed necessary for professional practice.

Thus, in a typical training session, the working position can be set up, the chair positioned for a specific treatment such as leg epilation, the epilation unit placed on the trolley and the necessary small equipment laid out in preparation for the task (see p. 32). This can then be followed by setting up the needle holder and epilation machine as if for use and conducting all the safety checks for good current connection.

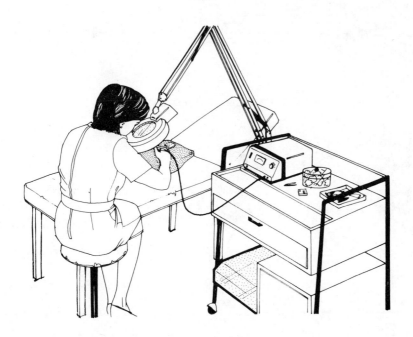

THE WORKING POSITION FOR PRACTICE

Preparing the Needle Holder
for Use

Where the needle holder and flex come apart, the needle holder should be wound down on to the flex to avoid stress on the more pliable area surrounding the wire connection point at the bottom of the needle holder. On the finger-control needle holders the button should then be checked and tightened if necessary as so to obtain a firm unrestricted 'tap' which will firmly connect the two metal strips inside the holder and allow the current to flow through to the needle. If the 'tap' is not decisive, the base of the button will not force the two strips to meet correctly, and this will result in a poor transmission of current, or no connection at all.

The new 'switch control' needle holders are a great improvement and eliminate these connection problems as the current is either *ON* with even the slightest finger pressure or *OFF* as pressure is released.

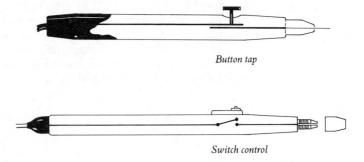

Button tap

Switch control

CROSS-SECTION OF NEEDLE HOLDERS

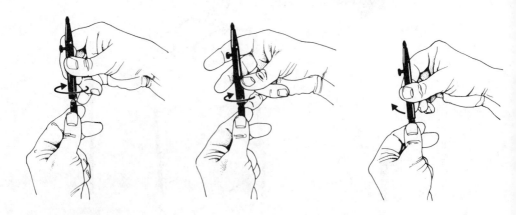

SCREWING THE MAIN BODY OF THE NEEDLE HOLDER DOWN TO THE FLEX

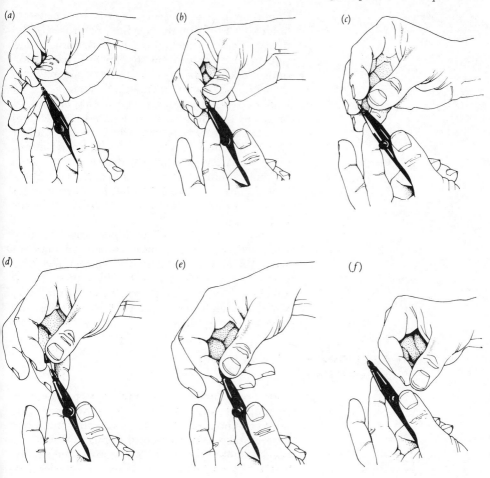

PREPARING THE NEEDLE INTO THE CHUCK

The covering cap of the chuck section should then be removed and the selected needle pushed carefully into place with the shoulders of the base shank just showing above the divided claws. If the connection is not firm, the needle should be removed and the claws tightened gently until no movement is evident when the needle is replaced. The cap can then be put back and the needle holder is ready for use. If the cap does not fit correctly, covering the metal of the chuck completely, it should be removed and the needle repositioned. Normally, in such instances, it will be found that the base of the needle has been pushed in too far, forcing the claws of the chuck too widely apart. If, therefore, the needle is gently pulled out sufficiently for the shoulders of the needle shank to show clearly, the cap will fit correctly. It is important that all the metal parts of the needle holder, apart from the needle, are protected by plastic coating which also covers the holder and cap, in order to prevent the current from being transmitted to these metal parts and possibly causing burns to the operator's fingers.

In between treatments, the needle should be protected by a soft plastic cover, and at the end of the day's treatments the whole needle holder should be removed from the machine and put in a place of safety—the trolley drawer or a closed container. Some machines have a special fitment in which to place the needle holder when it is not in use to protect it and prevent it falling from the trolley.

With practice, the needle holder can be set up and checked in a few minutes, and an operator who has become used to the correct feel of a perfectly functioning holder will soon notice if anything is wrong and will know straightaway where to look for faults and poor connections, and how to remedy them.

Safety Checks on the Epilation Unit

Before commencing an epilation treatment or training practice, several safety checks should be made to ensure a safe, effective and continuous performance. Starting with the epilation machine, checks should be made for good connections: firstly, by ensuring that the needle-holder flex

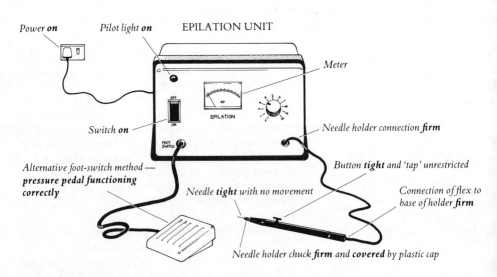

*Power **on***   *Pilot light **on***   EPILATION UNIT

Meter

*Switch **on***

*Needle holder connection **firm***

*Alternative foot-switch method — **pressure pedal functioning correctly***

*Button **tight** and 'tap' unrestricted*

*Needle **tight** with no movement*

*Connection of flex to base of holder **firm***

*Needle holder chuck **firm** and **covered** by plastic cap*

SAFETY CHECKS

connects firmly into the socket on the machine and that the connection plug is firmly screwed on; secondly, that the flex is tightened on to the base of the needle holder (a common cause of poor current transfer); thirdly, that the button is firm and taps clearly (if a button-type is in use); and, lastly, that the needle is firm in the chuck and the correct amount of needle is protruding. Then, apart from connecting the power supply from the wall socket and switching on the epilation machine, the unit is ready for use.

If, during the epilation treatment, the performance of the machine and the results obtained seem to be doubtful, the machine should be switched off and the above safety checks made. In addition, the intensity control knob, the mains power supply socket and the on/off switch should be checked, as faults can occur here as well.

The checking routine should start at the wall socket, continue through the controls on the machine, pass methodically through the connections of the needle holder and finish by testing the needle on a piece of damp cotton-wool.

PRACTICAL STEPS IN EPILATION TRAINING

Hand Movements

Competence in handling the small tools should be established at the outset, prior to applying the treatment to a client, so that later on full concentration can be given to the task of actually probing the follicle. The hand movements required for the probing and hair removal sequence can be practised, using a pillow to represent the 'client'. The

(a) Position   *(b) Probe*   *(c) Tap*

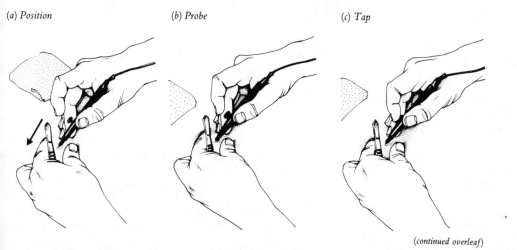

(continued overleaf)

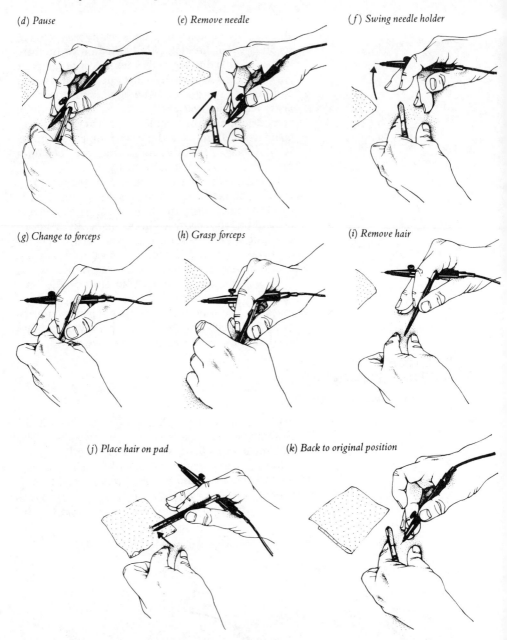

(d) Pause *(e) Remove needle* *(f) Swing needle holder*

(g) Change to forceps *(h) Grasp forceps* *(i) Remove hair*

(j) Place hair on pad *(k) Back to original position*

HAND CHANGEOVER ROUTINE—SEQUENCE OF MOVEMENTS (a)–(k)

changeover of the needle holder and forceps in the operator's hands can be practised until a smoothness of movement is achieved and the tools feel comfortable and balanced. Unnecessary hand movements should be kept to a minimum to increase the safety, speed and efficiency of the removals. Attention should be given to holding the needle point steady at the moment when the current would be connected, whether the connection is made by the button tap or through firm pressure on the foot-switch. This 'mock-up' of the routine makes it possible to introduce the short wave diathermy current into the routine later on with the minimum of disruption.

Probing without Current

As soon as the rhythm and balance of the tools in the changeover sequence are established, a simulated application on easily visible leg hairs can be undertaken, but still *without* using the current. This stage starts to develop the operator's sense of touch in probing the follicle and ability to sense when the base of the follicle has been reached. The need to align the probe with the angle of the follicle and to practise smooth, painless probing is also established at this stage. Firm holding and stretching of the skin to aid the needle probe's entry into the follicle develops alongside the probing skill.

If all these elements become established before the electrologist needs to be concerned with the additional problem of the client's reaction to the pain caused by the current application, confidence and skill can grow quickly in preparation for the next stage of the technique. This ability to probe the follicle gently and accurately, while holding and controlling the skin firmly but without distortion, is of vital importance to the electrologist's skill. Later, when undertaking really difficult probes, in highly sensitive areas, her skin handling and probing abilities will stand her in good stead and allow full concentration on the task in hand. For, if an electrologist is still uncomfortable or ill at ease with the use of her tools and the positioning of her fingers when she commences the epilation sequence, she may never conquer the nerve-racking task of inflicting pain (however slight) on another person.

When the tools feel comfortable in the hand and the operator is able to hold the needle point steady at the moment when the current would be connected, probing practice may commence on leg hairs.

Once the leg epilation working position has been set up, probing commences on the mid-calf area, to the side of the shin. Here, the probe angles are the easiest to follow, and the area can be reached easily by the operator without difficult hand or body positioning, thus allowing her to concentrate on the probes. The complete hand

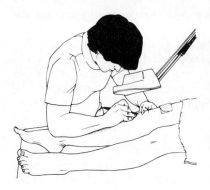

HAND POSITION FOR LEG
EPILATION

changeover sequence should be practised again, as if the current were actually being applied, and the dead hair removed on to the pad of cotton wool. Special attention should be paid to keeping the needle point steady both at the moment when the current would be applied and directly afterwards, in order to avoid pain and damage.

The operator should work in a comfortable position, with her back straight and not bent over. The height of the stool should be adjusted until the operator is able to reach the treatment area easily and without strain. Then the trolley and equipment should be positioned on the electrologist's working side (depending on whether she is right- or left-handed), so that the flex does not trail across the client. Students should not commence work until they feel comfortable in the working position and do not need to fidget and reposition themselves during the application. Unsatisfactory or uncomfortable positioning often results in inaccurate probing of the follicles as well as damage to needle holders and needles.

It has been observed that hairs grow at an angle to the skin, and the shaft, or free section, follows the contours of the body. On the lower leg, the hairs contour away from the shin, normally downwards towards the ankle at the lower (or distal) end and backwards towards the back (or posterior surface) of the leg in the calf area. This is most easily seen if the hairs are a reasonable length. Short hairs which have regrown after shaving or removal by depilatory creams give much less indication of their true angle under the skin. The section of the shaft closest to the hair's entry into the skin gives the operator guidance as to the likely angle of the hair root underneath the

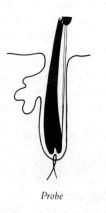

Probe

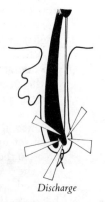

Discharge

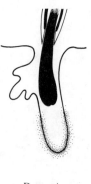

Destruction

CORRECT PROBE POSITION

surface. The true angles are quickly evident once probing actually commences, because, unless the angle of the hair in the follicle and the angle of the needle probe match up exactly, the needle will not enter the follicle easily and the probe will hurt the client.

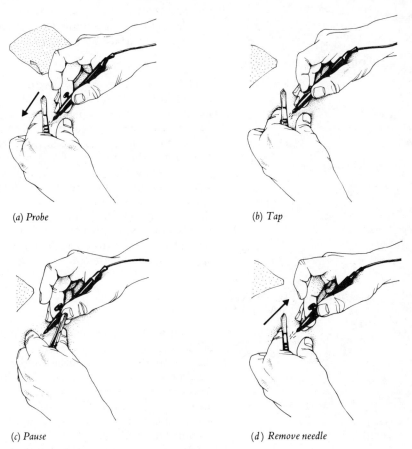

(a) Probe

(b) Tap

(c) Pause

(d) Remove needle

TAPPING AND PROBING SEQUENCE

Stretching the skin slightly in the early stages of learning the technique helps to allow the needle to enter the mouth of the follicle, but, unless the probe is positioned correctly, the needle cannot pass down between the hair and the follicle wall painlessly. At this stage, the trainee should concentrate on skin handling, stretching and probing techniques in order to become accustomed to the feel of the client's skin tissues, their resilience and their resistance to the finger pressure required to keep the skin steady. On the button-connection needle holders, special attention should be given to tapping firmly and smoothly, without movement at the needle tip or unnecessary repositioning of the fingers to accomplish the tap. The stages of the sequence should be practised with distinct pauses, for example: position—probe—tap—pause—remove needle—change to forceps—remove hair—back to original position. These pauses get lost in the epilation technique as speed increases, but are necessary initially to prevent the needle point moving while the current is flowing and causing surface burns.

Connecting the Current

Once the probe can be accomplished without discomfort and the needle held steady at the moment of current connection, actual hair destruction and removal can start. As all the steps to this point have been practised right from the start of training, the only things left to be incorporated into the sequence are choosing the current intensity to suit the hair strength, switching on the epilation unit and connecting the power supply at the wall socket. A sequence of safety checking measures to ensure that the unit and needle holder are functioning correctly is the last step before the application is undertaken.

COMMON PROBING FAULTS

So far we have seen that the essential ingredients of successful removal are accuracy in getting the current to the correct place in the follicle, and steadiness of hand to contain the current to the required area in order to prevent unnecessary damage to the skin. The *steadiness of the hand* is very important as the desired destructive effect cannot be produced if the chosen amount of current does not reach the dermal papilla matrix area. There are a number of points to watch for here:

(1) Movement of the needle may cause too much current to seep through to surrounding skin tissues leaving too little to accomplish the cauterization of the active hair root area.

(2) If the current is discharged above, below, or to the side of the active germinative area, again destruction will not take place and skin damage will result.

(3) The fine needles used may quite easily pass through the follicle walls or the base of the follicle, thus making the probe completely inaccurate. Only the operator's sense of touch and the client's reaction give guidance as to the accuracy of the probe.

Moreover, the correct *amount of current* must be discharged in order to obtain complete hair destruction. Often, although the correct intensity level is chosen to accomplish the epilation of a hair, the power of the current is lost through indefinite connection. This may be because of hesitation in operating the button tap or foot-

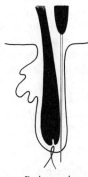

Probe too deep
INCORRECT PROBING

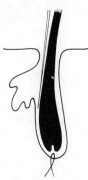

Probe too shallow

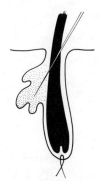

Probe into the sebaceous gland opening

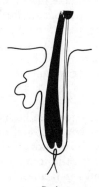

Probe
CORRECT PROBING

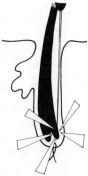

Discharge

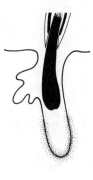

Destruction

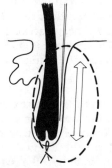

Up and down movement of needle— partial destruction; skin damage
INCORRECT PROBING

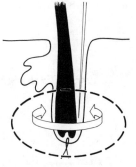

Shaking side to side movement— little effect on active area; large area of skin damage

switch, movement of the needle at the moment of current application, or because the needle is withdrawn too fast from the follicle after the application, thus preventing the diathermy current from completing the cautery of the matrix area.

It is only by actually epilating a hair, adding into the sequence the use of the current application, that one thoroughly understands that only the *correct amount of current*, discharged in the *correct position*, for the *correct length of time* will bring about *complete hair destruction* and, furthermore, that when the hair has been correctly epilated, it will be disengaged from the follicle and can be freely removed *without pulling*.

If, after the application, the hair cannot be lifted free without resistance, several factors need consideration before the hair is re-treated, as follows.

Accuracy of the Probe

First, was the probe sufficiently accurate to ensure that the needle point reached the correct position at the base of the follicle to allow cauterization of the tissues to take place? With the variation in follicle depths that occurs due to the hair growth cycle, so the probe depth must vary to reach the dermal papilla area. The electrologist's sense of touch will serve here to indicate when the base of the follicle has been reached.

Current Connection

Secondly, has there been a good enough current connection to allow the current to flow through to the needle tip? If the button tap or foot pressure has not been distinct and decisive, the connection may have only been partial or may in fact not have been made at all. In either case, the proper current flow would not have occurred. It is possible that no short wave diathermy current at all may have reached the needle. This would be evident from the fact that the skin at the mouth of the follicle would show no signs of normal heat reaction (erythema—skin reddening). The electronic switch control needle holder solves many of these problems.

Current Discharge

Thirdly, has sufficient destructive power (intensity or amount of short wave diathermy current) been available to complete the hair destruction satisfactorily, based on the diameter of the hair and its location? In training, the safer, lower-slower system of current choice will make it necessary to work with low intensities applied for fractionally longer periods in order to provide the necessary total amount of current needed to bring about the destruction. As long as the correct amount of current has been applied—by whichever method—the hair epilation will be successfully completed.

Needle Movement

Lastly, has movement occurred at the needle point at the actual moment of current application, thus dissipating the current and dispersing the destructive power into surrounding tissues? This, apart from causing excessive skin reaction, results in only partial destruction of the hair root, and the hair remains firmly attached to the follicle at its lower end and cannot be lifted free.

Other Factors

There are many other reasons why hairs are not successfully removed, some associated with distortion of the follicle or abnormally active growth, others concerned with the location of the hair and the hormonal influence governing its growth and distribution. These abnormalities will be studied in later chapters, but need not concern the trainee in the early stages of acquiring practical skills. In practice sessions, the work is concentrated on normal hairs which follow a normal growth cycle, and the probing errors considered are the most common causes of failure in the early stages of acquiring practical technique.

DETERMINATION OF FAULTS BY OBSERVATION OF HAIR AND SKIN

Close observation of the skin and the hair during and after the epilation application will assist greatly in achieving a successful technique. Real accuracy in hair destruction can only be seen to have occurred if either the hair does not regrow at all, or regrows, but in a modified form, as a regrowth-type hair.

If a correctly epilated hair (one that comes freely and without resistance from the follicle after treatment) is removed by forceps and placed on the cotton-wool pad, it can be studied closely and will be seen to have a fully formed root structure with tissue sheaths intact if epilated at the *anagen* stage of growth, or a club-like root structure if epilated in *catagen* or while in transition prior to being shed.

The root structure may have become damaged in the cauterizing process and may not have an

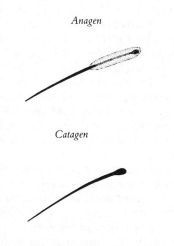

Anagen

Catagen

CORRECTLY EPILATED HAIRS

intact root, but, if it lifts freely from the follicle the chances of successful removal are good. Only the non-appearance of a new hair or the presence of a regrowth hair will tell how effective the first application has been in destroying the follicle's capacity to re-form a new hair. This effect of destroying the growth capacity of the follicle is of greater importance than the actual removal of the existing hair.

After treatment, the hair often remains firmly attached to the follicle. The operator should not be tempted to tug the hair out, as this is pointless and painful for the client. If, despite several attempts to epilate the hair, it remains firmly connected to the follicle, the basic causes of failure, as outlined above, have to be considered. The most common fault in the trainee is the **dislike of applying the current firmly**, allowing the current to flow and complete the destruction, because it causes pain to which the client reacts. It is, perhaps, the hardest and most unnerving aspect of electrology for the student to master. It should be remembered that clients with a genuine hair problem are prepared to put up with some discomfort to achieve the solution to their problem, and, in order for the operator to resolve the unwanted hair condition, she has to use the short wave diathermy current effectively and allow it to do its work. Her indecision does not help the client attain the results she seeks, but leads rather to frustration and disappointment.

If the hair is seen on removal to have broken off along the shaft and to be without the root structure, then it can be concluded that the **current has been discharged too shallowly** within the follicle, destroying the hair shaft, but not affecting the root or matrix area. The follicle will then form another hair of identical strength to the original, although it may be distorted due to the damage that has been done to the follicle. This can occur if the needle enters the opening of the sebaceous gland at the upper end of the follicle, through poor positioning, rather than following the true angle of the follicle and hair. Normally severe skin reaction will occur in association with this probing fault.

If, during the application, the skin around the mouth of the follicle becomes excessively red, or white and inflamed, it may be an indication that a **surface burn**, which immediately after the application will appear as a white swollen ring, has occurred. This suggests the current is being discharged too close to the surface, or that the needle

Probe into sebaceous gland causing severe reaction and surface burns

SKIN DAMAGE

is being moved at the moment of application of the current. Shaky hands or unsteadiness will cause the needle to move, allowing current to escape to the drier surface skin layers and cause a surface burn. The client's instinctive movement away from the sensation is also a factor to be taken into account here. Unless the operator's confidence has developed prior to this stage and she is prepared for this, a chain reaction may occur in which the client jumps, which makes the operator jump and unnerves her, which in turn makes her hand move, thereby causing current spillage and a burn to occur. Some electrologists believe that less needle movement occurs when using a foot-switch connection because the hand is then freed from the need to move to tap the button. However, many things can cause needle movement, even the repositioning of the body as the foot pedal of the unit is depressed to connect the current, and only practice and awareness of the hazards of needle movement can eliminate the problem.

Another problem in technique that can be observed when studying the skin is **excessive use of current**. This is different from too little use of current in that it actually does destroy the hair, but it also damages the skin unduly. Following the initial **surface burn** and white ring reaction, the skin forms scabs at the mouth of the follicle. This can lead to depigmentation (loss of skin colour—or white patches), scarring and hyperpigmentation (red or brown patches). Even if the skin does heal and recover without permanent injury, the time taken for healing to take place slows the treatment sequence. This is less of a problem with leg hairs because these are well spaced, and the skin is able to stand up to the effects of treatment without too many long-term effects. But, in any area of densely placed hairs, such as around the lips and chin, over-treatment might occur on converging areas, and this would not only slow the progress of the treatment plan while healing took place, but would also cause permanent disfigurement, pitting, marking, discoloration and damaged skin texture.

It is for this reason that all initial practice takes place on the leg hairs, these being easy to see and probe (having clear, well-defined probing angles), while being spaced far enough apart to permit the skin to recover without permanent injury. This allows the trainee electrologist to progress to the next stage without losing confidence, or too many friends or clients.

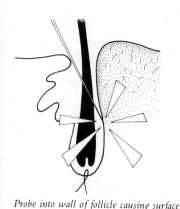

Probe into wall of follicle causing surface burns and possible capillary damage

SKIN DAMAGE

Indeed, getting past this initial stage in gaining technique is a major hurdle, but, once mastered, the trainee has the requisite skills to progress to more difficult, interesting and rewarding work. Most practice will be undertaken on fellow students as it is very valuable to gain first hand experience of the sensation of epilation and to appreciate its discomfort personally. This creates sympathy for clients' feelings and a wish to minimize their discomfort which spurs the trainee on to improve her probing technique and handling abilities. Once the early nervousness has been dispelled, then suitable clients can be introduced to the practice sessions to help the students build up confidence and speed from more extended periods of work. One of the best ways to establish technique and build confidence is to work quietly with a suitable client, uninterrupted for a long period, until the pace of the work becomes rhythmical and the rate of removals increases steadily. In this way the operator learns to correct her own mistakes, rather than always relying on the lecturer for help.

ASSESSMENT OF CURRENT INTENSITY

We have seen that successful removal of an unwanted hair relies on the electrologist's skill in probing and discharging the current accurately. It also relies on her skill in assessing the amount or intensity of current that must be applied and the appropriate length of time. The judgement depends on several factors, *most important of which is the capacity of the skin physically to stand the diathermy application.* The diameter of thickness of the hair, its nature (horny, curly, etc.) and its location are other considerations, but it is the restriction imposed by the sensitivity of the skin which is the vital factor.

Sensitivity of the Skin

The sensitivity and healing capacity of the skin itself determines the course of progress by limiting the amount of epilation that may be applied and dictating the periods between treatment on any one area. Its healing and recovering powers can, however, be improved with good clinical procedures. Special precare and aftercare skin treatments, including the use of ozone vapour steaming to promote healing, can be used which will extend the amount of work that can be carried out. Meticulous attention to technique will also ensure that the skin does not become overtreated and liable to damage and scarring.

Client's Pain Threshold

The ability of the client to bear the discomfort is another major consideration in successful electrology. Skins have varying capacities to withstand the cauterizing effects of the diathermy application, and equally diverse are individuals' capacities for pain. The pain threshold, as it is often described, dictates the intensity of short wave diathermy that can be applied and the overall duration of the applications. Naturally this varies acording to the area to be treated, some areas being far more sensitive than others, owing to their nerve supplies and other factors.

Nevertheless, the client's tolerance to epilation can be improved by sympathetic handling which will help to put her at ease and instil confidence about the task ahead and its successful outcome (see Chapter 4).

Nature of the Hair Growth

A further consideration in determining the correct current intensity is the nature of the individual hairs themselves—whether they are fine or coarse, straight or curly, or have been previously subjected to other hair removal remedies. Another factor to be considered is the hormonal influence which results in the growth of particularly resistant hairs (see Chapter 5).

Thus the hair itself, its nature, its location and the client's skin and pain capacity all play a part in determining the intensity and duration of current necessary for epilation to be successful and yet to avoid skin damage. The advantages of the different methods of application—either low and slow or high and fast—become clear as experience grows. They provide for all skin conditions, pain thresholds and hair strengths. The lower intensities are very suitable for the trainee, until accuracy and client handling skills develop with both methods; however, the *total* amount of short wave diathermy current applied is that which is necessary to accomplish the hair destruction without skin damage.

If attention to technique is accurate, and the hair still remains firmly attached to the hair follicle, either the current level can be increased fractionally, or its application extended a fraction of a second on the subsequent application. If the operator is nervous, the fault is commonly associated with loss of current through needle movement or poor connection due to anxiety not to hurt the client. Correction of these problems often provides a solution to the failure of the hair removal, and increased intensity of current or prolonged application of current is not needed—simply more accuracy and confidence.

REGROWTH

Normal Superfluous Hair

Most superfluous hairs require only a fractional amount of short wave diathermy current to destroy them and render the follicles ineffective, and hairs of weak growth, if accurately treated, will not regrow. However, if limitations of the current intensity due to skin sensitivity or poor healing prevent complete destruction from being accomplished, regrowth will result. The modified regrown hair can be subsequently dealt with when it reappears and a successful result achieved. Regrowth will be inevitable if hairs grow from abnormally active follicles and are resistant to treatment, and this should be borne in mind when treatment is planned.

Effect of Abnormal Hormone Imbalance

Abnormal hormonal imbalance or steroid therapy may make regrowth more persistent and medical guidance should obviously be sought in cases where response to treatment is disappointing. It is preferable for both the client and the operator to be fully aware of the magnitude of the problem and the treatment necessary to achieve good long-term results, even if there are inherent difficulties. The operator can then plan accurately, alter her technique accordingly, and can support and encourage her client in resolving her hair problems.

Effect of Previous Treatment

Any previous treatment will also affect the rate of regrowth that can be expected, as any distortion of the follicle naturally affects the accuracy of the probe and can prevent the current being discharged at the active matrix area because traditional needle probes are not suited to distorted or curved follicles. Results will be far slower on hairs that have been persistently plucked or waxed prior to epilation than on untouched or virgin hairs, or those which have simply been cut off. The hairs which emerge as a result of plucking are also often confused with true epilation regrowth hairs, appearing as they do as much as six to eight weeks after being plucked. This is why it is important to ask the client not to pluck hairs in the treatment area once a treatment programme has commenced, but to cut or even shave them off if she wants to retain a clear appearance.

The operator can learn a lot in early training from assessing the regrowth from treated follicles, and should follow clients' progress on clinic record cards to see how her technique, and results, are improving. For *hairs removed* often does not correspond with *hairs destroyed*, which is the whole purpose of the treatment.

In the hands of the trainee, insufficient current is one of the main causes of failure to detach a hair and for regrowth problems. This caution is natural enough when client discomfort is involved, and can be remedied by slowly increasing current intensity until just the necessary amount of current is obtained and no more.

Leg hairs which are mainly used for practice in the early stages of establishing technique are *normal* strong hairs, which require quite a high level of current intensity to remove them. So, for the trainee these are ideal, in that they force the operator to be decisive in her choice and application of the current strength, otherwise the hairs remain very firmly attached. In addition, the trainee will be able to see that to remove even strong, normally active leg hairs, only a fraction of a second of current application is needed if the current has been chosen correctly and applied smoothly and decisively. On many machines only an intensity of 1½ to 2, or for exceptionally strong hairs perhaps 3, on the intensity control, applied for a fraction of a second (via button tap or foot-switch), effectively destroys the follicle's capacity for regrowth, and the hair can be lifted free. When one considers that this has been accomplished by employing the low-slow method, it becomes apparent how little current is actually necessary to provide destruction if it is applied accurately within the follicle. So client discomfort should never be severe, and should decrease progressively as the operator's technique and skill grow.

TREATMENT OF LEG HAIRS—PRACTICAL PROGRESSION

Once the first hurdle of successfully removing a hair has been overcome, and the operator has developed the ability to judge the current intensity needed for hair destruction, then the application can be organized into a treatment. Treatment details must be recorded to avoid overtreatment and, to prevent skin damage while technique is improving, the actual applications must be well spaced in order to allow the skin to recover and to avoid skin marking.

The working position is prepared and the client made comfortable, with the area of the leg to be treated clearly in the operator's view and accessible to her hands. Paper sheeting may be used under the client's legs for comfort and hygiene. Basic details may be recorded on the client's record card at this time and added to when the treatment has been completed. The skin area—initially mid-leg—is then wiped over with a cleansing and cooling lotion, *following the direction of the hair growth*, and epilation can commence. The epilation unit having been set up and checked as previously described, the intensity control is returned to zero, and, after inspection of the hairs, the intensity level is set ready for use. This safety procedure prevents any possibility of the intensity control being used at an incorrect level and must become an *automatic* step. This awareness of the machine and its intensity level is also important when a variety of different hair diameters are treated within one application session, and the intensity or amount of current used has to be consciously altered on the unit. This is done in preference to prolonging the application or tap on the button or foot-switch, which is the more common way to increase or decrease the amount of current applied when working on very similar hairs in an area.

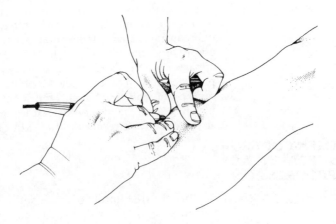

NORMAL PROBE ANGLE

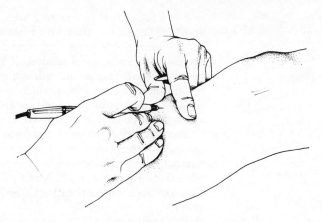

ANGLED PROBE: FIRM HOLDING AND STRETCHING

Mid-leg Area

In the mid-leg area, the operator's hand holds the needle holder much like a pen, and the probes are normally deeply angled into the skin, as if pointing to the inner core of the leg. The position of the hand and probe alters according to the area of the mid-leg treated, with some probes being almost upright.

Ankle Area

On the lower leg the hairs lie flat, shallowly placed along under the skin, and, as less subcutaneous flesh is present, the probes are more difficult. In addition, the epilation application is more sharply felt in this area, thus increasing the client's discomfort. So, treatment has to be plan-

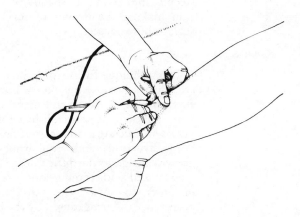

ANKLE PROBE: FINGERS EXTENDED

ned carefully in this sensitive area, working for short periods at a time, then moving away to more comfortable areas and returning at a later stage or at a subsequent session. If a client finds a treatment unbearable, she will not persevere with it, and therefore a method which will provide the desired results, while recognizing the client's pain limits must be devised during treatment planning.

The flat positioning of the hairs requires the operator to position her probe at an angle almost parallel to the skin and to hold the needle holder with the fingers extended. Many of the probes in the ankle area will be pointing directly towards the knee.

The button tapping method requires the index finger to remain free to connect the current, although the actual supports of the needle holder, the thumb and middle finger, remain the same, opposing each other, to hold the needle holder steady and position it. Probes in the ankle area are undertaken carefully, and should not be undertaken until competence is reached on mid-leg hairs.

In order to work on the ankle, the operator must reposition herself and, therefore, she becomes accustomed to working at different positions and altering the magnifier, her own body posture and the client's position to make accurate work possible. This flexibility will be valuable later when undertaking epilation on awkward areas, and will help to maintain a good technique. Practice in working with an extended hand position on the ankle while maintaining control of the small tools is valuable preparation for more difficult work on the inside thigh, abdominal area, throat and facial areas. Here the probes are often steeply angled and lie shallowly along under the skin making the danger of severe reaction and surface burns acute.

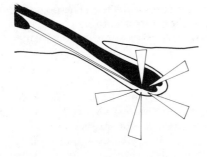

STEEPLY ANGLED ANKLE HAIRS:
CURRENT SEEPAGE

Knee Area

The technique for treating the hairs of the knee area differs because the skin is horny, difficult to enter and probe well, and many of the hairs are very shallow and of a club-hair formation. It is a very sensitive area, and lack of flesh, closeness of bony structures and stubbornness of the hair growth all add to the difficulties. The skin must be well soaked with cooling lotion prior to epilation in order to soften the skin and prevent the occurrence of burns caused by the horny nature of the skin. The lotion must also be used generously during the application to soothe and settle the skin and reduce client discomfort. Firm holding and stretching permit the follicle to be probed. As with the ankle area, only short sessions should be attempted, interspersed with work in other areas.

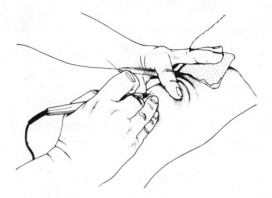

PROBING ON THE KNEE AREA

The probe angle on the knee is very upright and almost directly towards the middle or centre of the knee. This is a very tiring probe angle for the operator and again this is excellent hand practice for other difficult areas which have the same, almost upright, follicle direction—for instance between the brows, on the backs of the fingers and toes, and occasionally on the breast bone area in breast hair treatment. Also, in many instances the hairs are very superficially placed, requiring great control to avoid superficial burns, white ringing or the formation of scabbing rings. For this reason practice on knees is invaluable, and although marking and scarring does occur, the skin can recover without permanent injury or scars.

Front and Back Thigh Areas

The client is made comfortable in a semi-reclining position for work on the front of the thighs, and a prone position for the back thigh area. Pillow supports can be used to prevent the client getting a stiff back from sitting in one position, and also to make her more relaxed and comfortable while the treatment is carried out.

Hairs on the front of the thighs can be treated in approximately the same way as mid-calf hairs, being similar in character and probe direction. The legs can remain resting directly on the couch, not lifted or supported by pillows, but rather positioned by the operator to enable her to probe the area easily.

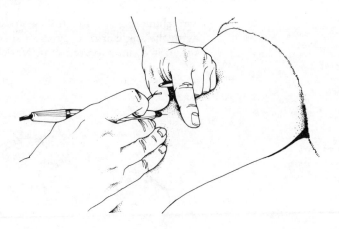

FRONT THIGH

The increased fleshiness of the thigh calls for increased stretching and holding away of the skin tissues from the immediate treatment area to allow the probe to be accomplished and the needle to enter the follicle painlessly. Fractionally increased intensities of current strength are also required to accomplish a successful removal in this area because the soft tissues appear to absorb the current, leaving less available to complete the hair follicle destruction.

Hairs on the back of the thighs have to be examined very closely to ascertain the probing direction as they have a tendency to swirl round in a growth pattern quite different from that of the

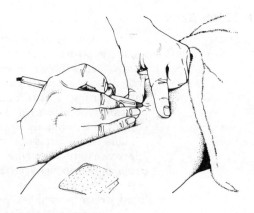

BACK THIGH

front of the thighs. Close attention must be paid to the direction of growth of each individual hair, rather than assuming that many of the hairs will grow in a similar direction. Every care should be taken to see that the client is as relaxed as possible, and that back strain is not adding to her discomfort and overall tension. Increased relaxation can raise the client's pain threshold and thus a great deal more work can be accomplished in the same period of time.

Inside Thigh Area

The inside thigh is a highly sensitive treatment area, and the client must be positioned carefully to permit probing to be accomplished accurately. The hairs are often extremely strong and coarse in nature, being basically pubic hairs which have overgrown their normal position due to a general hairiness of the client. As the hairs' natural direction is downwards and backwards, it is sensible to treat them by probing towards the base of the follicles, which involves working from the opposite side of the client. This avoids the necessity of having to work with the hand position reversed, an operation which is both very difficult for a trainee, and not very accurate.

The thigh to be treated can be supported on a pillow and protected with a towel or paper sheeting, not only to provide modesty for the client but also a hygiene barrier for the operator who inevitably must come into contact with the client as she works across her.

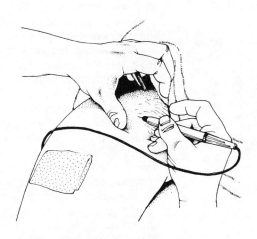

INSIDE THIGH

Most of the probes in the inside thigh area are steeply angled into the skin, and a very flat probe is necessary, using the extended finger position. Each hair follicle must be probed very carefully otherwise the hairs will remain firmly attached, and the epilation application will be extremely painful for the client. The probe follows the hair follicle, entering the follicle mouth then flattening to progress down the follicle to its base. This is a special technique which calls for *extra care* rather than any extra skill. The hairs in this area are often stubborn, and, if initial probes are not successful in removing the hairs, they should be left and treated at a later session. The skin in this area quickly becomes irritated, red and sore, and so the probes should be well spaced and special precare and aftercare measures taken to avoid infection of the follicles. The client should be advised to avoid underwear rubbing the area after treatment and to wear loose fitting garments to prevent additional discomfort.

On removal, some of the strongest hairs will produce blood spot formations, which look unpleasant, but are simply a result of the current intensity used and the vascular nature of the area, and will quickly disappear. Clients should, however, be advised of this occurrence to prevent anxiety.

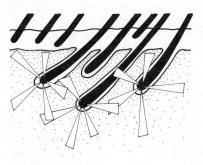

STEEPLY ANGLED HAIRS:
CONVERGING HEAT REACTIONS

THE ABDOMINAL AREA

The client should lie flat on the couch, as close to the edge as possible, with a pillow to support her head and tissue protection above and below the treatment area. The magnifier should be positioned on the opposite side of the client from the operator to allow space for the epilation to be applied, as the direction of the probes in this area may vary considerably. In some instances the operator may even need to stand to complete a particularly difficult probe.

Hairs in this area are of two main types—the hairs which are pubic in type following the body mid-line in an upwards direction and those which surround the umbilical area or belly button in a circular fashion and which may be either fine in texture or also strong pubic-type hairs. Following the direction of each hair accurately is vital, and guidance can be obtained by observing the natural direction of the hairs as they leave the follicle. Care should be taken to wipe the skin with the preparatory cooling lotion *only* in the direction in

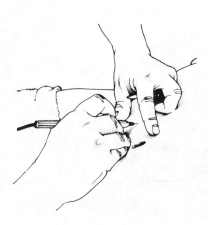

PROBING ON THE
ABDOMINAL AREA

which the hairs grow, otherwise it will be difficult to determine the likely follicle direction under the skin. Work on the abdominal area is one of the most difficult in which to achieve successful removals, mainly because of the variety of the probe angles, stubbornness of the growth and softness of the skin. Extremely firm skin holding and stretching is necessary to enable the needle to enter the follicle, and care should be taken not to lean on the needle or bend it in an attempt to achieve follicle entry. *Force will never accomplish a good probe, only accurate repositioning.*

The diameter of the needle used depends mainly on the type and thickness of hairs to be treated, but a needle of medium diameter—a Ferrie needle of .004 diameter—may prove the most satisfactory in this soft skinned area. It is not so much that the hairs themselves are resistant to removal in the area, but rather that it is difficult to position and hold the needle holder steady while the epilation application is completed. Many hairs fail to become detached due to loss of current through needle movement or inaccurate probing (as mentioned previously in Common Probing Faults).

Practice in this difficult area is invaluable in establishing hand control, probe accuracy and handling techniques on soft areas of the body. The same precare and aftercare measures, and the same generous use of soothing lotions during the treatment as is used during treatment on the inside thigh area, will all help the client's capacity to bear the application. These measures will also help to reduce any harmful effects of the treatment—erythema (skin reddening and increased skin temperature), soreness or infection, skin spotting, scabs or depigmentation.

Treatment for both abdominal and inside thigh areas should be of short duration. Clients can seldom cope with more than half an hour of treatment in these areas, normally less. Electrologists should work at the pace which suits the client's capacity and pain threshold, even if this reduces the number of removals accomplished. Disregard of the client's feelings in this matter will be bad for business.

FACIAL EPILATION

Once competence has been attained in the various aspects of leg and body technique, the operator is ready to tackle facial epilation with confidence in her technical abilities and skill in client handling. Facial epilation is no more difficult in terms of the probes to be accomplished, but the risks to the client from skin damage and scarring, for instance, are more acute, and so it is essential to have mastered most of the technical problems before commencing work on the facial area.

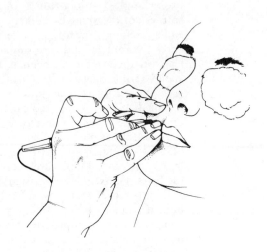

FACIAL EPILATION

A very important factor to remember when working on the face is that it is extremely sensitive, and the electrologist may well find the client's reaction to the discomfort very distressing. The facial area becomes progressively more sensitive as you move from chin and throat area towards the lips, with the area under the nose being the most painful because branches of the lower facial nerve are in close proximity to the upper lip area. Reactions to epilation in this area may include tears in the eyes, sneezing and twitching in addition to normal discomfort reactions such as pulling away and jumping, so the operator must be prepared for this and be in full control of her tools in order to avoid errors caused by these sudden movements.

For facial epilation, the client should be either in a semi-reclining or nearly upright position on the couch, depending on the area to be treated. If only a flat treatment plinth or massage couch is available, the client can be brought into a good working position with pillow supports, but the operator may need to stand to complete her work.

The operator positions herself in front of the client, close to her, and the magnifier is extended from behind the client. The operator's stool can then be adjusted to permit easy access to the client's facial area. The close position of the operator, tucked in tight to the client, also provides a feeling of reassurance for the individual as well as enabling the operator to sense the client's reactions through the physical contact. The epilation unit is positioned on the operator's working side and within easy reach to allow any minute current adjustments to be made without repositioning.

Facial epilation practice should commence on easily visible hairs on the chin area, not only because they are the easiest to probe and remove, but also because the skin is less susceptible to surface burns and bad reactions. The area should be inspected carefully prior to cleansing to determine the hair and skin condition. Skin cleansing milk may then be used to remove any make-up and, after thorough removal with moist cotton-wool pads, epilation lotion can be used to prepare the area. The reaction observed during the gentle cleansing and wiping sequence will help the operator in her assessment of the skin's sensitivity, and aid her in treatment planning. The skin is left clean and moist for the epilation application, but should not be wet, otherwise the operator will find hand positioning difficult.

The probe angles are very varied in this area, and as the hairs may be very short, having been previously removed by the client, it is sometimes difficult to assess the follicle directions. The hand position must alter according to the probe direction, and the operator may well find herself having to use all her fingers to accomplish the probes without hurting the client or distorting her features. Firm but gentle skin handling is needed, and roughness should be avoided at all costs. The operator's control over her hands and tools will really show up at this stage of practice. The client's eyes may be covered by cotton-wool pads to protect her from the glare of the magnifier, but these should be shaped so that they do not interfere with the work being carried out.

Chin Area

The hairs on the chin are often influenced by hormonal activity and may be strong in character and abnormal in growth, thus proving difficult to remove permanently. The first few probes should concentrate on getting the probe depth correct and ascertaining the ideal current intensity level to accomplish hair destruction without skin damage. Initially, the operator should work with a low intensity level and increase it gradually until the

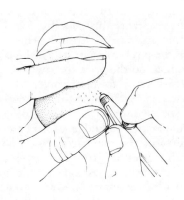

ESTABLISHING PROBE
DEPTH CAREFULLY

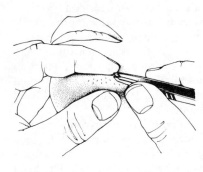

HOLDING SKIN TO AID
REMOVAL WITH FORCEPS

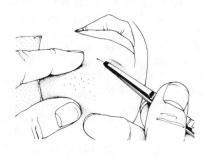

INSPECTING HAIR TO ASCERTAIN
CORRECT PROBE DEPTH

required level or amount of current is reached. Care in these first few probes establishes the follicle depth and guides the operator in her removal technique so that she can achieve hair destruction with the very minimum use of current, thus preserving the skin texture. Inspection of the first few hairs epilated will establish the growth pattern encountered, and help the operator in her treatment planning.

Abnormally active growth, distorted follicles, etc., will tell the operator what rate of progress to expect and how much regrowth will be forthcoming. Skin reactions should also be closely watched in the first few moments of treatment to establish the maximum amount of short wave diathermy current that can be used. Excessive skin reddening, white ringing, swelling, and so on all indicate errors in technique or the wrong current intensity level. Hairs should be epilated with due regard for the skin's sensitivity, which, as has been seen, *must* act as the limiting factor in determining current intensity.

In the case of *strong* superfluous chin hairs, the intensity of the current used may be sufficient to detach the hair, but not to destroy its growth potential. So a regrowth hair will appear, easily distinguishable from the original hair, and this can be treated at subsequent treatment sessions. Incidence of regrowth should be recorded in order to provide a comprehensive guide to overall progress. As technique and accuracy increase in facial hair epilation, the incidence of regrowth will decrease, and this will also give a good guide to the operator's progress.

At this stage, it is advisable for the trainee to perform *all* the treatments necessary on a client and to keep an accurate and continuous record. This will greatly assist the assessment, not only of the client's progress, but also of the operator's work. In this way, skin reactions, scabbing, infected follicles and so on, if they occur, can be analysed, and the technique corrected to avoid any recurrence. Only in this way can the operator's technique really advance in readiness for lip hair removals, where surface burns, excessive use of current and other similar problems pose a real threat to the client's appearance and well-being.

Hairs on the chin are very varied in character, angle, diameter, colour, texture, etc., depending on the reason for their growth. In some cases the tissue sheaths have become excessively thickened, filling the follicle cavity completely and making probing and needle entry difficult. Here, fine strong needles, good skin holding and stretching and very accurate probing—angled exactly to the direction of the hair—are essential.

On the chin area, the hair often grows densely, concentrated into two areas either side of the jaw, below the mouth. This means that the hairs have to be cleared gradually, and complete removal is not usually possible immediately as the areas of skin affected would converge, making skin healing slow. Where the hair growth is closely packed, some treatment organization has to be established to avoid over-treatment or skin damage. Careful records must be kept of the exact area of treatment, when it was performed, the results obtained, any skin reactions noticed, as well as the exact needle diameters used, the current intensities used and the epilation unit used to carry out the work.

Naturally, really full details of each treatment cannot be kept because the work on the face is so varied, even within one treatment session. However, basic details entered on the client's card do help to prevent mistakes, especially in training, and are valuable when treatments are performed by a number of operators. Students should be encouraged to discuss the client's condition and learn from each other's experience regarding skin sensitivity, probe angles and special problems dealing with the growth.

Professional treatment sessions for chin hairs are normally a quarter or half an hour in length, often combining both lip and chin hair epilation if the problem affects both areas. A trainee, working slowly and carefully, will possibly take twice as long to complete the same number of removals as a professional electrologist. Although professional speeds must be attained prior to obtaining commercial work, initially accuracy is far more important, than speed. For it is *hairs destroyed* not *hairs removed* that is important, and professional speed grows very quickly once epilation is practised every day.

Aftercare of the epilated area includes use of soothing, anti-inflammatory lotions to calm the skin and promote healing. This is followed by the use of flesh coloured, antiseptic powder or cream where necessary to disguise the erythema and protect the skin from infection, bacterial invasion, etc. (see Chapter 4). Clients must be advised about home aftercare and dissuaded from interfering with the hair growth between treatments, apart from cutting the offending hairs that remain. They should also be advised against cutting hairs just prior to their next appointment and thus leaving the operator nothing to treat.

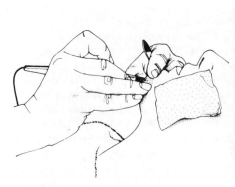
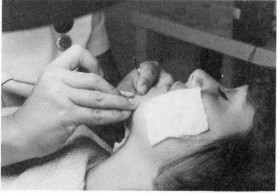

Chin epilation; point of chin

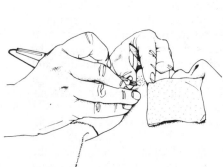
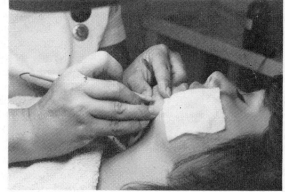

Side chin; close-packed hair formation

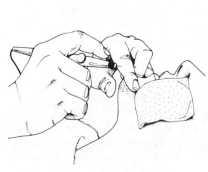
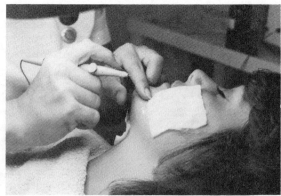

Removal, keeping finger in place to pinpoint treated hair

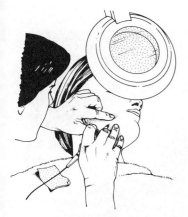

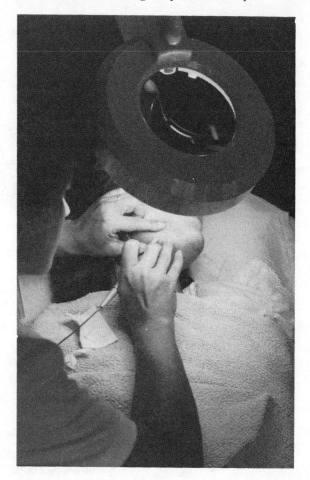

Probing on mandible (jawline), different finger position (more distant view)

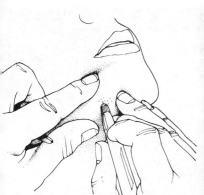

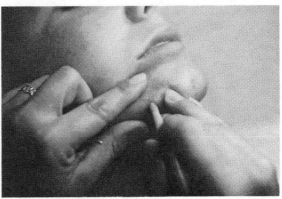

Close up of probe on side chin/mandible area

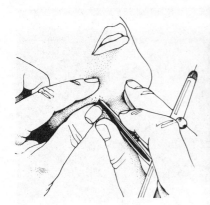
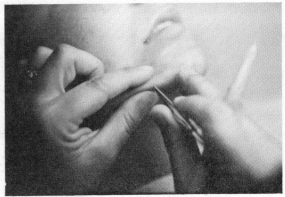

Removal, showing skin rolling to present the short hair for removal

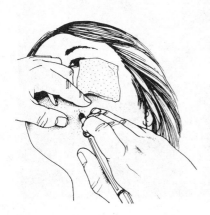
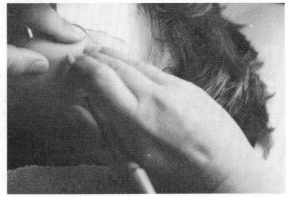

Probe on below-jaw area, using fingers in three-way stretch to bring hair into accessible probe angle position

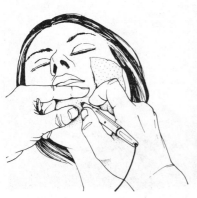
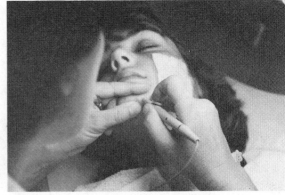

Work on abnormal growth needs to be well spaced to avoid skin damage

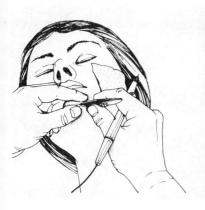
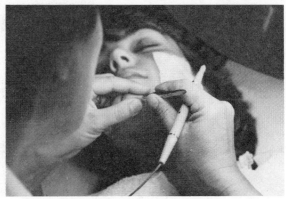

Hairs must lift free without resistance

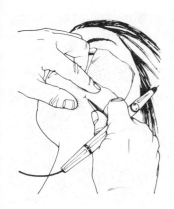
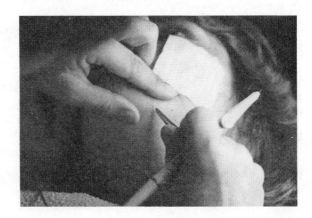

Skin resistance indicates that hair requires further treatment, and must not be 'pulled' out

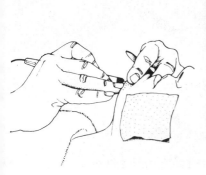
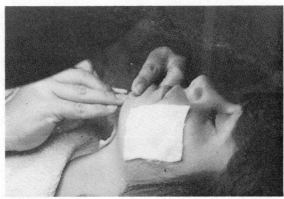

The ring finger can be used to steady the probe, and help skin stretching

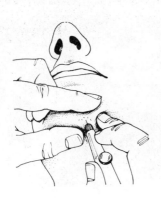
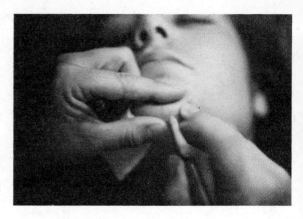

The skin can be 'bunched' slightly by the supporting fingers, to present very short, beard-type hairs for probing

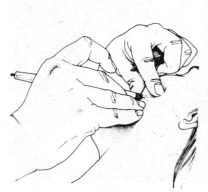
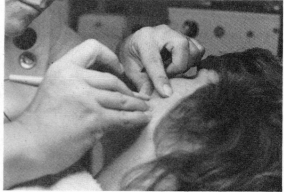

Abnormal hairs on the cheek must be probed carefully and slowly, as they may have very deep follicles, and abnormal growth

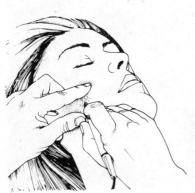
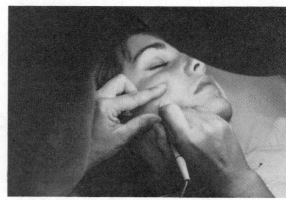

Long cheek hairs often have a very flat probe angle

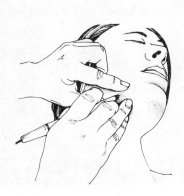
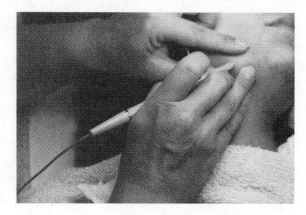

Alternative finger holding for jawline probe

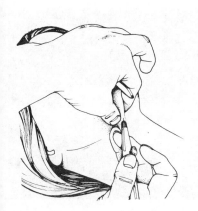
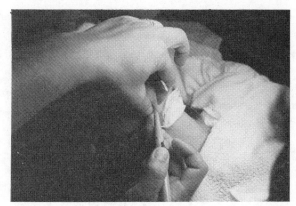

Probing on the neck, head reclined, neck relaxed, fingers used to roll and bunch the skin to make the difficult probe possible

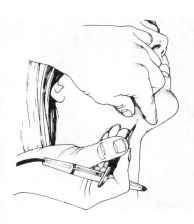
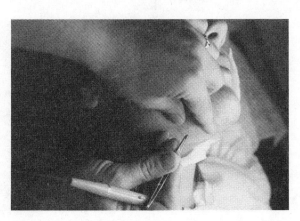

A correctly epilated hair; the softness of the skin often makes a perfect removal difficult

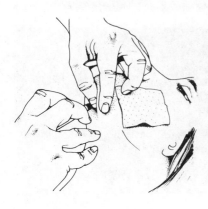
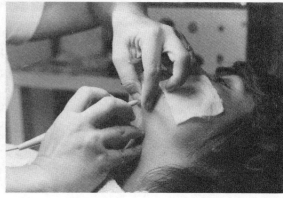

Picking up the skin gently for a difficult jawline probe

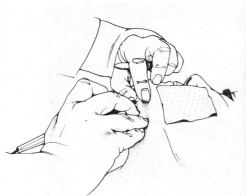
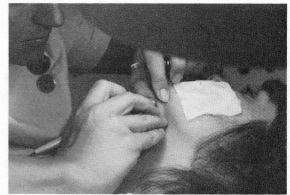

The operator needs free movement of her arms to complete some difficult probes without resting on the client

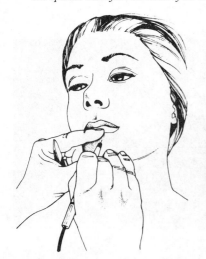
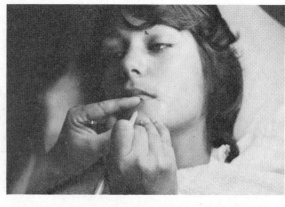

Hairs in the chin fold can be probed more easily if the skin is stretched upwards, and steadied along the jaw

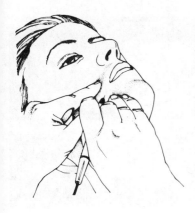

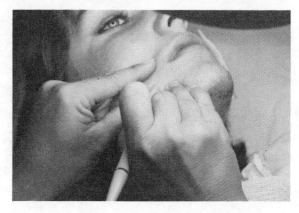

Stretching and steadying for a side lip probe

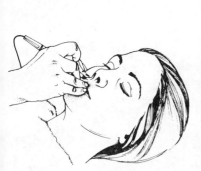

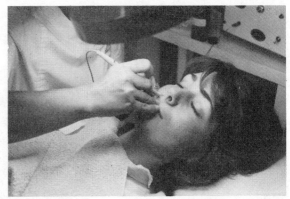

Upper lip probes with very gentle skin handling and control

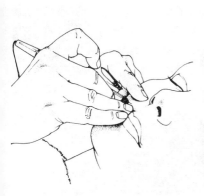

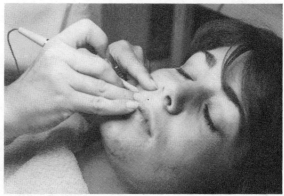

Meticulous attention to the probe angle is necessary on the lip

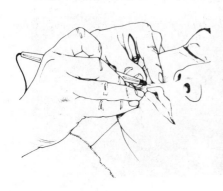
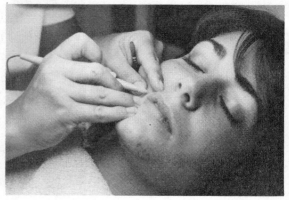

In previous untouched hairs, the probe angles are often similar on the side lip, angled towards the nose

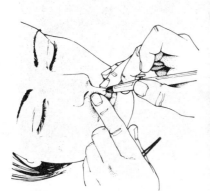
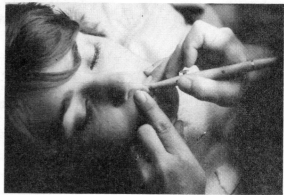

Pushing the skin together under the nose, to allow the probe to be accomplished

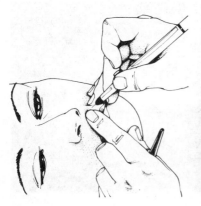
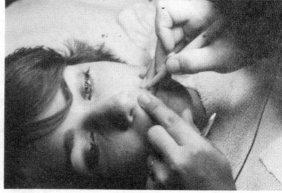

Bunching of the skin, or stretching techniques may prove most useful in the sensitive lip area, depending on the angle of the hair

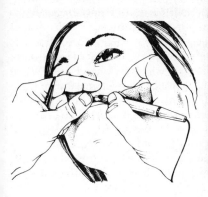 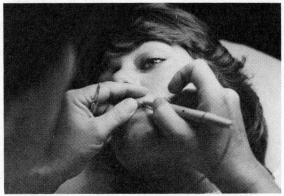

Hairs on the lip line need very careful skin holding while probing

Upper Lip Area

This is the most difficult area because of its sensitive nature which results in possibly considerable client discomfort. Nevertheless, the lip area relies on exactly the same techniques as all other aspects of electrology. Here, however, all skills have to be applied with particular diligence, although previous experience should permit the electrologist to progress to operating in this area without too much trauma for either herself or the client.

Initially, confidence can be built by working on easily probed, visible hairs. Once this has been mastered, fine, shallowly placed hairs can be tackled. A wide variety of needle diameters—from .003 to .005 in diameter—will be used depending on follicle size, hair diameter or thickness, skin sensitivity and so on. Most facial epilation can be accomplished with a Ferrie steel needle of .004 diameter, as this combines strength with fineness and is sufficiently flexible for most applications. The insulated, or German needle, which by virtue of its extra length is rather more difficult to handle, will also be used once probing skills grow. It is only available widely in one diameter, normally equivalent to .004, which is found satisfactory for most facial hair conditions. The special advantages of the insulated needle in restricting surface reaction makes it particularly suitable in cases of hypersensitive skin and problem cases. The new rounded-probe insulated steel needle is now available in diameters from .003 to .006 and these are invaluable for facial work.

Lip hairs have several growth patterns depending on the factors which caused them. If the hairs are basically a normal growth on a rather hairy individual, excessive but not abnormal for them, the hair growth will be quite straightforward to treat and will respond well showing results quickly. This is especially true if the hair problem has not been interfered with, but is in its virgin state, having never been plucked or waxed out. When the hairs are well spaced, complete clearance of an area is possible, as long as the hairs treated are one-tenth to one-eighth of an inch apart (2 to 3mm) at least. Trainees should work in a well-spaced, chequered fashion to avoid converging skin reactions which could cause swelling and slow healing, thus holding up further work. If the hairs are well spaced, epilation can progress from the outside area of the hair growth inwards, so that the hairs can be selected, probed and removed easily, thereby improving the rate of removals. The use of angled forceps helps to prevent the picking up of untreated hairs growing alongside the treated ones.

If the growth is of a very dense, but fine nature, possibly the result of hormonal influence, then care must be taken to avoid skin damage as a result of the superficial placing of the hair roots. Surface burns and skin damage from converging areas of treatment must be avoided by careful treatment planning. Fine Ferrie needles can be used, in some instances as fine as .002 or .003 in diameter, and the current applied very carefully to avoid spillage and burning of the drier, horny surface tissues. The hairs seem to be sitting almost on the surface of the skin, hardly in it, and probing is very tiring on both the operator's hand and eyes. It can be almost impossible to see fair hairs of this type entering the skin, and the magnifier must be positioned to throw light down on to the hairs to make them stand out, rather than directly on to them, which seems to make them disappear.

It should be remembered that this type of vellus growth comes from normal follicles prompted into greater activity through internal stimulus— for instance, natural hormonal fluctuations such as pregnancy, or perhaps artificial stimulation such as the Pill. As a result, the hairs can be very difficult to remove completely, especially if the hormonal stimulation is still taking place. Even though the hairs are basically fine, the internal influences affecting their growth are strong, and regrowth can be quite a problem. The client's awareness of the background factors relating to her hair problem help her understanding of the treatment problems, and, therefore, client discussion is vital in this instance.

The horny type of hair growth which often comes as a result of the menopause is extremely common, and will make up a large percentage of the professional electrologist's practice. Hormonal influences are again at work, but the process is a natural one, and unwanted hair growth can be considered alongside many other signs of ageing as a natural, if unwanted, sign of getting older. As the female hormones lose their dominance, male hormones become less restricted, and in the middle-aged woman a common result is the formation of unwanted hair, often in the male sexual pattern in severe cases. The upper lip, chin and occasionally the throat and cheeks are involved, with follicles changing in nature to produce horny hairs out of character with the more normal vellus growth. Hormonal influences use the normal vellus hair follicle as a vehicle for this strong hair growth, but only specific areas are sensitive to this influence. It is extremely unusual to find unwanted hair in the menopausal client in areas outside those mentioned. This acts as a guide to the operator in planning her treatment programme and points to a successful outcome to the treatment.

The hairs may have suffered from a considerable amount of prior treatment by temporary removal methods such as plucking, waxing or depilatories and clients will often be very surprised by the true number of hairs present which are not initially visible. Careful recording of the hair condition at the first consultation is important in establishing the fact that *additional* hairs have become evident in the early weeks of treatment, thus preventing any dissatisfaction with the results on the part of the client. Discussion at an early stage can avoid any confusion over this point.

Previously treated hairs may have distorted follicles, which, although they are not particularly difficult to probe, suffer from a far higher degree of regrowth, thereby making results slower. Really strong individual hairs may be treated first to bring about an immediate improvement in appearance, and a high level of current intensity may be needed to destroy them. Being deeply placed in the skin, the danger of surface burns is not as great, but, because of the intensity of current that has had to be applied, the probes should be well spaced.

Its important to aim at achieving an immediate improvement in appearance to encourage the client and prevent her feeling tempted to pluck out offending hairs. Some sympathy for the client's situation is necessary, and solutions should be suggested to retain a reasonable appearance while treatment is in progress. Certain areas can be left for epilation treatment and the remainder cleared by temporary methods, cutting being the least destructive to the skin. If a growth is very heavy and extremely fast growing, the hairs can be removed between treatments by depilatory creams as long as the skin is accustomed to the effects of the chemicals used and does not become sensitive or easily irritated. Use of depilatories can cause increased skin reaction to the epilation treatment, thus slowing down progress.

Treatment of strong and fine hairs can be interspersed within any one treatment session by altering the current intensity and possibly the needle diameter as well. This will extend the client's capacity for treatment, and provides rests from the more painful applications. Just as the operator can 'rest' certain areas of the lip by moving around with her probes, so she can rest the client by working on different types of growth, thereby varying the level of discomfort. In a small area such as the upper lip, it is very easy to over-treat the skin, and the operator must be on the alert for this and immediately alter her technique or halt the treatment. The skin's capacity for epilation can be extended by liberal use of soothing, anti-inflammatory lotions during treatment. These reduce swelling, settle the skin and reduce skin trauma and reaction.

Once areas have been treated, they can be covered with moist, thin cotton-wool pads soaked in lotion, which adhere to the skin and reduce its colour and heat. Treatment can then progress to adjacent areas, leaving the cotton-wool pads in place, already starting the healing process.

This care in treatment will reduce the need for camouflage measures after the application, as the skin will regain its normal colour and can then be easily covered by medicated powder or cream. Thus, the client will be less tempted to apply make-up in the affected area, which could result in skin infection.

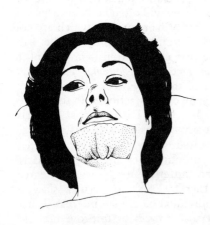

CLIENT AFTER TREATMENT

Chapter 3

Detailed Study of the Skin and Hair

In order to complete her work safely and effectively, the electrologist must have a thorough knowledge of the structure and function of the skin and the hairs which lie within it. Later, the forces which control the growth of the hair will be considered (see Chapter 5). But, initially, the formation, structure and functioning of normal follicles within the skin are of greater relevance to practical techniques.

This intimate knowledge of the histology of the skin and hair provides the key to the reversal of the hair growth process, and permits follicle destruction without skin damage.

STRUCTURE OF THE SKIN

The skin is made up of two layers: the **epidermis**, or outer covering, and the **dermis**, or true skin, beneath which is a layer of **subcutaneous fat**.

The diagram of the skin shown here demonstrates the relative anatomical positioning and gives a clear indication of important areas for consideration by the student of electrology.

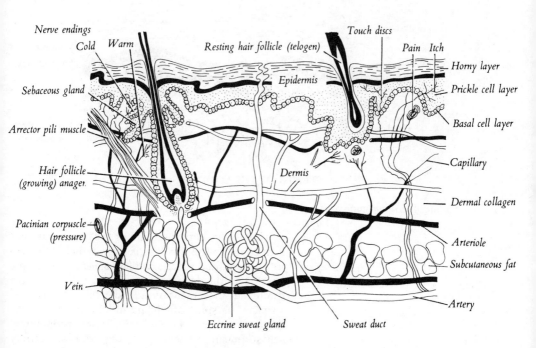

SKIN STRUCTURE

The Epidermis

The outermost part of the epidermis consists of flat, dead cells that are constantly being worn away or shed. The underlying part is made up of rapidly dividing cells which are continually pushing upwards and replacing the dead cells above them. Consequently, the layers of the epidermis represent every stage from basal cells with well-defined nuclei to superficial debris in which all evidence of cell structure has disappeared.

The epidermis has five layers grouped into two main divisions:

STRATUM CORNEUM

Stratum corneum, a dead horny layer;
Stratum lucidum, a clear hyaline layer;
Stratum granulosum, a layer with cells which acquire keratohyaline granules.

LIVING STRATUM MALPIGHII

Stratum spinosum, a prickle cell layer;
Stratum germinativum (or basal layer), a living layer, where mitotic activity (cell division) takes place.

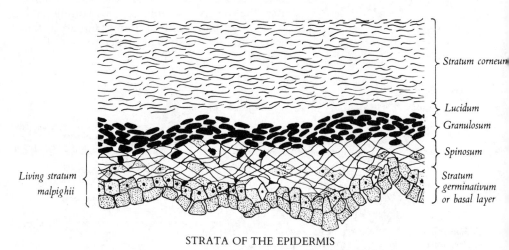

Living stratum malpighii

Stratum corneum

Lucidum
Granulosum

Spinosum

Stratum germinativum or basal layer

STRATA OF THE EPIDERMIS

Stratum Germinativum or Basal Layer

This is the deepest section of the epidermis, and is in contact with the dermis from which it derives its nutrient fluid via the *capillary blood vessels*. In the basal layer the development of new cells leads to a gradual displacement of the older cells towards the surface. In spite of apparent low mitotic, cell-dividing activity, the epidermis is a reproductively self-sufficient system that regenerates entirely from cells resident within it.

Melanocytes, cells which form the pigment *melanin*, are found in abundance in the stratum germinativum—one in every ten cells being a melanocyte. Melanin protects the skin against injury from ultraviolet radiation, and is responsible for differences in skin coloration. Melanin is formed from the amino-acid tyrosine by a complicated series of chemical reactions. The dendrites (branches) of melanocytes are in contact with at least one basal or Malpighian layer cell, and they are the only cells capable of forming and distributing melanin in the epidermis. Melanocytes seem to share the fate of Malpighian cells, being desquamated or shed off in scales at the surface of the skin.

Stratum Spinosum

The prickle cell layer is often classed with the stratum germinativum, to form the basal layer. Most mitotic cells which appear to be in this spinous layer are actually found in the basal cells around the dermal papillae of the hair in other layers, and mitotic activity takes place largely, if not entirely, in the stratum germinativum. The prickle cells are well-defined polygonal cells, and the whole layer is connected organically by means of the prickle-like threads which join up the cells.

Stratum Granulosum or Granular Layer

The thickness of this layer may vary from one to several cells' depth and is thickest on the palms of the hands and soles of the feet. The cells are flattened, and evidence of granules of keratohyaline may be seen if the skin is stained. These cells reflect light and give the skin a white appearance.

Keratinization is the change of living cells into dead, horny, flat cells with no nucleus. Fluid loss is an essential process in the stages of keratinization, and the stratum granulosum cells are believed to represent the first stage in the transformation of the epidermal cells into the horny material, keratin.

Stratum Lucidum

This layer derives its name from its clear translucent, almost transparent, appearance. It is only a few cells deep and lies between the outer horny layer and inner granular layer. It is thought that the stratum lucidum is the site of the barrier zone controlling the transmission of water through the skin. At this level of their growth towards the surface, the cells have lost their clear-cut line, and the nuclei are becoming indistinct.

Stratum Corneum

The superficial portion of this horny layer contains mainly layers of dead, flattened, keratinized cells, which are constantly being shed. The cells contain an epidermal fatty material, which keeps them waterproof and helps prevent the skin cracking and becoming open to bacterial invasion. This surface layer forms the greater part of the thickness of the epidermis in many parts of the body. Nuclei are no longer evident here, cell structure has become completely obscured, and, from below upwards, the flattened remains of cells become gradually converted into cornified flakes. The stratum corneum is crossed by the ducts of sweat glands and by hairs where they are present.

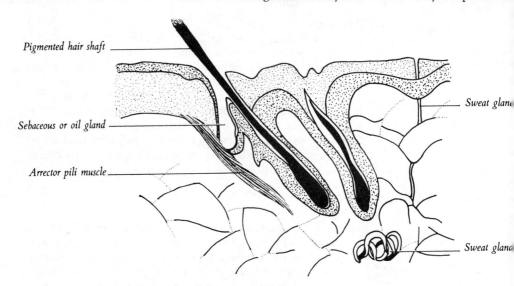

Pigmented hair shaft

Sebaceous or oil gland

Arrector pili muscle

Sweat gland

Sweat gland

DIAGRAM OF HAIR, SWEAT AND SEBACEOUS GLAND

The epidermis rests upon the dermis, a dense fibrous layer beneath it, into which it interlocks by a series of finger-like projections called papillae. The irregularity of the basal layer of the epidermis can be clearly seen from the diagram.

The Dermis

Being a condensed connective tissue, the dermis is unstable and undergoes change, breakdown and renewal. The dermis contains elastic tissue, blood vessels, lymphatics, nerves, tactile corpuscles and hair follicles, and is totally different in structure from the epidermis. The dermis is thicker in men than in women, and thicker on the *dorsal* and *extensory* surfaces of the extremities than on the *ventral* and *flexor* areas of the same individual. It is thickest on the palms and soles of the feet, but, being continuous with the layer of subcutaneous fat, it lacks exact boundaries and its thickness cannot be measured accurately. The dermis has a superficial papillary layer and a deep reticular layer.

Papillary Layer

In the papillary layer, widely separated, delicate, collagenous (gelantinous), elastic and reticular fibres, enmeshed with superficial capillaries, are surrounded by abundant, viscous ground substances. The surface of the layer is shaped into intricate valleys, ridges and papillae, while the cutaneous appendages (hairs, etc.) that extend into the dermis, piercing the reticular layer, are accompanied by the papillary layer throughout their length. Around hair follicles, the papillary layer forms the connective tissue sheath.

Reticular Layer

The fibrous reticular layer is composed of dense, coarse, branching, collagenous fibre bundles, which form layers mostly parallel to the surface. A few fibres can be traced down to the subcutaneous fat layer, subcutanea, where they branch loosely, becoming incorporated into its framework, and form the *retinacula cutis* that separate the fat into lobules. Loose networks of elastic fibres between the collagenous fibres are more closely woven around the cutaneous appendages. Around the blood vessels and nerves, the connective tissue fibres are always delicate and more widely spaced than they are elsewhere. Connective tissue cells, more of them in the papillary layer than in the reticular layer, are sparsely distributed among the fibres.

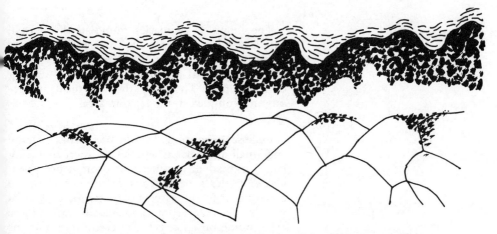

NORMAL SKIN WITH WELL-DEVELOPED PAPILLARY PROCESSES

Cutaneous Blood Vessels

The thickness of the skin, the types and numbers of cutaneous appendages present, the relationship of the skin to the underlying muscle or bone, and many other factors, all influence the vascularity of the skin and the form the blood vessels take in the area.

ARTERIES

The arteries to the skin anastomose (join and branch) below the hypodermis, where they form a large, meshed 'facial network'. Arterial branches from this network traverse, or cross, the hypodermis across the retinacula cutis and divide again in the lower limits of the dermis. A second, large-meshed, 'sub-dermal', ill-defined arterial network, parallel to the deeper one, is formed at this level. Above this level, no pattern of vascular vessels is clear, since the entire dermis is riddled by a continuous meshwork of branching arterioles and capillaries.

ARTERIOLES

Some arterioles seem to run a fairly straight course through the dermis, and branch in tree-like fashion underneath the epidermis. Hair follicles are accompanied along their length by blood vessels, running parallel to them. These vessels are still interconnected by arteriolar and capillary cross-shunts (valves) and anastomoses to the main vascular network. The straight portions of the ducts of eccrine sweat glands are also accompanied by similarly longitudinal-positioned, interconnected arterioles and capillaries, which at the level of the papillary body become connected with the intricate plexus (network) of the vessels there.

CAPILLARY LOOPS

The loops of capillaries found in the dermal papillary ridges between the epidermal ridges are most numerous in regions where the underside of the epidermis has the greatest amount of ridging or sculpturing. Therefore, they are most numerous and complex in the friction areas.

VENULES

In close association with the meshwork of large and small arterioles is a series of interconnecting large and small venules. A prominent *venous plexus* in the subcutaneous tissue is even more extensive than the associated network of arterial vessels. Between venous and *arterial plexuses* there are numerous direct inter-communications through which blood is shunted, so passing into the venous circulation without having to traverse the capillaries. In other words it bypasses them.

The complex and often apparently chaotic distribution of vessels in the dermis is nevertheless well adapted to the various changes and stresses to which the skin is exposed. The major vessels, being convoluted or snake-like in structure, allow a distension or stretching of the skin without appreciably interfering with the circulation of blood. This adaptability is particularly evident during the various phases of the hair growth cycles. In catagen, for example, the hair follicle withdraws upwards, leaving the lower part of the follicular vascular basket collapsed below it. When the follicles become active again, they must force their way through these collapsed vessels.

The venules in the skin have a remarkable ability to contract and dilate, in comparison with those in other tissues. Blood can be shunted through arterial venous anastomoses directly to muscular venules, omitting the various lateral capillary networks. The increase in blood through these shunts does not increase the diffusion from blood to tissue. Rather, these shunts are important for the regulation of blood pressure, and act as safety valves. Rises in blood pressure from *vasoconstriction* (constriction of vascular vessels) opens the shunts automatically, thus preventing excessive rise in pressure.

Temperature regulation is the main function of cutaneous vessels, but the function of pressure regulation is also very important.

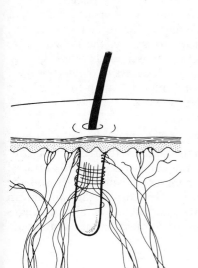

VENOUS SUPPLY TO THE SKIN

Nerves of the Skin

CUTANEOUS SENSORY NERVES

Our standard concept of the distribution of the cutaneous sensory nerves is that there is a *deep cutaneous plexus* in the *panniculus adiposus*, from which tortuous fibres cross the dermis to the papillary body, where they form a *superficial cutaneous nerve plexus*, less complex than the deep one. Many fibres from the deep plexus are also thought to go directly to the papillary ridges of the epidermis. A *third plexus* just underneath the dermo-epidermal junction is said to form large, irregular meshes.

Cutaneous sensory nerves have a simple basic pattern. The nerve fibres of the *neurons* in the *dorsal root ganglia* come together in the dermis, where they form intricate, interconnected **networks**. A stimulus applied at any point on the skin evokes not one, but a pattern of responses. Since this network of fibres is present in all skin, it is probably its principal sensory **end organ**. There are no end organs found in the mucous membrane, only a network of nerve fibres.

NERVE NETWORK

During development, the nerve network is the first ordered structure to appear in the dermis, and may influence the development of cutaneous appendages. The plan of the dermal nerve networks varies with the density of the cutaneous appendages. In regions heavily populated with hair follicles, we find few cutaneous sensory nerves, but, where follicles are sparse, the networks are prominent. Smooth muscle, sebaceous glands, sweat glands and the thickness of the dermis itself all have a profound influence upon the particular form of the nerve networks.

END ORGANS

Specialized, encapsulated end organs are found only underneath the glabrous (hairless), cutaneous and muco-cutaneous epidermis which has a ridged underside. The number of hair follicles and the number of specialized endings in the skin are, in fact, in inverse ratio to each other. Skin perceives so many different forms of sensation that it would

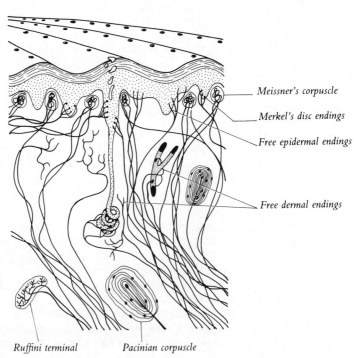

Meissner's corpuscle

Merkel's disc endings

Free epidermal endings

Free dermal endings

Ruffini terminal   Pacinian corpuscle

NERVOUS SUPPLY OF THE SKIN

be impossible for each of them to be served exclusively by an automatically distinct end organ. *Meissner corpuscles*, the *Hederiform ending*, and the *muco-cutaneous end organs*, all seem to be sensory endings for *acute* touch, but the *principal organ for the perception of touch must be the nerve network around the hair follicle.*

Temperature, pain and other sensations are perceived by a variety of different receptors. It would seem that the specialized end organs are modified according to the region in which they grow, and not according to the special function that they serve. The only specialized end organ for which a relationship to a specific sensation is known is the *Vater-Pacini corpuscle*. Stimulation of the end organ gives the sensation of pressure, but it does not send a signal to the receptor until a definite pressure threshold is reached.

Glands

SWEAT GLANDS

Sweat glands are tubular in nature and start their life in the deeper layers of the dermis. The coiled body of the gland opens onto the surface of the skin via a long narrow tube passing through the skin's layers. The sweat glands are divided into two types: the *eccrine* glands and the *apocrine* (or large coil) glands. The eccrine (or true sweat) glands secrete water and water-soluble substances and are found in abundance all over the body, apart from the margin of the lips and certain areas of the sex organs. The main function of the sweat glands is the regulation of body temperature by evaporation from the surface of the skin. The apocrine glands are connected to hair follicles and are found mainly in underarm, breast and genital areas of the body. They secrete cellular waste, fatty substances, water and salt. 'Body odour' is most closely connected with these glands, which are also thought to play a part in sexual attraction.

SEBACEOUS GLANDS

Most sebaceous glands are appendages of hair follicles and open inside the hair follicle cavity via a duct. The size of the gland often varies inversely with the size of the hair follicle with which it is associated. On the face, some very large glands, among smaller ones, empty into the dilated pilary canals of vellus (downy) hair follicles. Sebaceous glands are most numerous on the scalp, forehead, nose, chin and cheeks, and in decreasing numbers on the back, the rest of the trunk and the limbs. They are of epidermal origin but lie in the dermis forming irregular-shaped structures.

These glands secrete a fatty substance, *sebum*, which helps to keep the skin and hair supple, and plays a part in protection against bacteria. Sebum is markedly different from tissue fats, and a number of unusual substances not found elsewhere in the body can be detected in the sebaceous secretion. Cholesterol, free fatty acids and lipid products of keratinization have been traced in different quantities. The amount of sebaceous lipids on a particular area of skin could be dependent in part upon the number, size and rate of secretion of the glands, and the thickness and wetness of the skin.

The glands are influenced by the action of the endocrine system and, at puberty, become very active, often causing facial blemishes.

FUNCTIONS OF THE SKIN

The skin acts as a covering for the body, and it has four main functions although the first is the most important:
Protection;
Heat regulation and elimination;
Secretion and absorption;
Sensation.

Protection

The horny, outer layer of the skin, the stratum corneum, is tailored in every detail to protect the body against its environment. The structure, rate of replacement and physical repair properties of the outer layer protect against bacterial invasion and minor injury. The skin is waterproof and acts to contain body fluids while preventing the entry of large quantities of fluid through the epidermis.

Heat Regulation and Elimination

Loss of body heat is mainly controlled by the blood supply and sweat glands of the skin. Evaporation of sweat from the surface is an automatic process, which works efficiently unless the surrounding air is also hot and moist. The complex distribution of blood vessels in the dermis is well adapted to the various changes and stresses to which the skin is exposed. Body temperature regulation is the main function of cutaneous vessels, but blood pressure regulation is also important. Through dilation (expansion) of superficial capillaries, surface heat is lost and body temperature is reduced. The skin changes colour and appearance, becomes pink and warm and, combined with perspiration loss, reduces discomfort effectively. To retain heat, the blood vessels constrict (contract) and become smaller in diameter, and the passage of blood slows, giving a blue or dark red appearance due to loss of oxygen. The skin looks pale, and the *arrector pili* muscles can cause the hairs to stand erect in order to trap air close to the surface.

Secretion and Absorption

Sebaceous secretion, sebum and perspiration, helps to keep the skin supple and intact. Decomposed sebum and perspiration combined with bacteria produce 'body odour'. Considerable quantities of water are lost in perspiration as an automatic reflex action in body temperature regulation. As the prime function of the skin is protection, its absorption role is limited, although there are several routes through which agents may enter. The hair follicle and sebaceous gland opening, and the skin itself, are capable of absorption, as is the sweat duct to a lesser degree. Penetration is affected by the health and condition of the skin, and breaks or irregularities in the surface increase the risk of infection.

Sensation

The skin contains nerve endings which make us aware of our surroundings. They act as a warning system to indicate heat, cold, pain, pressure and other external factors. The nerve receptors are located at different levels in the skin, touch and pain indicators being close to the surface and closely involved with the reactions received from the hairs. Pacinian corpuscles, which indicate pressure, lie deeper in the skin, so that a certain threshold of pressure would have to be reached before sensation was stimulated. Cold indicators lie at varying depths beneath the surface, and, like other organized endings, are accompanied by pain receptors.

THE SKIN'S DEFENCE AGAINST BACTERIA

The normal skin is never sterile, its surface being contaminated by a wealth of bacteria. Most of these are non-pathogenic (not disease-producing) and cause neither harm nor inflammatory reaction. Other bacteria, such as *staphylococci* and *haemolytic streptococci*, which in certain circumstances can provoke inflammation, may also be present without exciting any reaction. In the course of its evolution the skin has come to accept many such organisms as part of its natural *resident* bacteria. It has the power of inhibiting or restricting their growth until a state of equilibrium has been reached. When this control fails, or *transient* bacteria become present, boils, folliculitis, or other skin disorders occur. An overwhelming invasion of organisms from some outside source, or a new and virulent strain, may precipitate such attacks. The mechanisms available to the skin to prevent or limit the invasion of these bacilli (bacteria) are numerous and complex. The most important factors are as follows.

Acid Mantle

The aqueous fluid bathing the outer surface of the skin is acidic in nature and acts as a defence mechanism against infection. It is known as the 'acid mantle'.

The pH (acidity) value of the horny layer in healthy skin ranges between 5 and 5.6, showing an acid reaction compared to a neutral pH of 7. The acid mantle is formed by the secretions resulting from the activities of the sebaceous and sweat glands, and the process known as keratinization of the epidermis. This mantle plays a most important role since it acts as a protection against action exerted by bacteria and micro-organisms living in the external environment, which is characterized by an alkaline pH. In addition to this, the acid mantle is a determinant factor in the maintenance of the healthy aspect of the skin surface. In fact, a decrease in acidity in the skin tissue results in an unhealthy appearance with uneven texture.

pH VALUE OF SKIN TISSUE

Cutaneous pH varies according to the different layers of the skin, thus the pH of the inner layer is similar to that of blood plasma, approximately 7.35, while in the outer epidermal strata it is between 4.8 and 5. Scientific research has revealed that the principal constituents of the acid mantle are represented by acid proteins. The physiological acidity and the pH of the skin tissues (5 to 5.6) may vary greatly, according to external and internal factors such as sunlight, beauty cosmetic applications, skin hygiene, digestion and nutrition, and may change within twenty-four hours. Excessive perspiration can also cause the pH to change. A 6.5 pH favours the development of micro-organisms, causing a number of dermatoses (skin disorders).

Fatty Substances

Sebum secreted from the sebaceous glands contains a complex mixture of lipids and fatty acids, some of which are bacteriostatic (growth inhibiting) and others bactericidal (destructive). Adult sebum is also fungicidal and can help prevent some types of ringworm. By keeping the surface of the skin smooth and free from cracks, abrasions, etc., the sebum plays an important part in maintaining an intact skin surface.

Sweat

The sweat exerts a powerful bactericidal effect: by maintaining the surface of the skin at a certain level of acidity it inhibits the growth of organisms. However, excessive perspiration decreases the acidity, and encourages the growth of bacteria while softening the skin's surface and thus making entry easier.

Horny Layer

The horny layer itself acts as a protection against invasion. Normally, it is impervious to fluids and bacteria, but its protective mechanisms can be damaged by caustic preparations and elements which alter oil, fluid and pH levels of the skin.

Desiccation

There is evidence that simple 'drying out' of bacteria limits their spread. The value of moderate applications of dusting powder can be seen in many skin conditions.

Vascular Reactions

If an organism manages to invade the main body of the epidermis, an inflammatory response is aroused. Histamine is liberated; vascular dilation, oedema and leucocytosis occur. The *leucocytes* engulf and destroy invading organisms as soon as they pierce the horny layer. The skin may react violently to the external agent in an attempt to prevent the spread of infection to surrounding tissues.

Thus, it can be seen that many of these mechanisms are mutually antagonistic. The integrity of the normal skin depends upon a balance between them. This protection against infection is remarkably efficient considering the abuses and injuries to which the skin is continually subjected.

KERATIN

The stratum granulosum is the *keratin-producing* layer, where *keratohyaline granules* are usually collected at the poles of the nucleus. They are specific products of epidermal cells, which become a part of the final horny component of cornified surface skin cells. Equally involved in the formation of the final horny component are *cytoplasmic fibrils*.

Loss of fluids is an essential process of the final stages of keratinization. Some dehydration of transforming cells starts at a distance from the skin's surface and at a level where normally hydrated cells also occur. Dehydration does not seem to be due to simple desiccation and evaporation of water. Loss of fluids at this level is probably caused by *syneresis* or some similar process through which the proteins release their water-bound molecules. At higher levels, closer to the surface, desiccation and evaporation of water may be at work, leading to complete consolidation of the cell content.

Two fundamental types of keratin, 'hard' and 'soft', are recognized.

Soft Keratin

Soft keratin is found in the epidermis, the internal root sheath of the hair follicle and the medulla of the hair. It is supple and pliable, has a moderate sulphur content and a high fluid (lipid) content, and is continuously desquamated or shed.

Hard Keratin

Hard keratin differs from soft keratin in its toughness and firmness, and in its permanence as it is not desquamated or shed. Hard keratin has a high sulphur and low fluid content, and within its structure there exists a *keratogenous zone*, which is a transitionary area between the basal (Malpighian) layer and surface, horny, keratinized layers. It is found in nails, the cortex and the cuticle of the hair.

MITOTIC ACTIVITY

In spite of apparent low mitotic (cell dividing) activity, the epidermis is a reproductively self-sufficient system that regenerates entirely from cells resident within it. Cell division in the epidermis occurs mainly in the basal layer. Most mitotic cells which appear to be in the spinous layer are actually found in the basal cells around the dermal papillae in other layers, and mitotic activity takes place largely, if not entirely, in the basal layer. This, therefore, is the *true stratum germinativum* of the epidermis. The rate of shedding (desquamation) and the rate of mitosis, or cellular division, in the epidermis relate closely to each other. It appears that growth exactly replaces loss most of the time.

During bodily activity the mitotic rate is low, and during sleep and rest it is high. Excessive muscular activity or exposure to extreme cold are followed by a nearly complete depression of the mitotic rate. Both adrenaline and cortisone have a powerful antimitotic action, which possibly works by interfering with carbohydrate metabolism, or the way food is used by the body to fill its needs. Thyroxine also decreases mitotic activity, while testosterone increases it. Such fluctuations in the mitotic rate are, however, relatively minor variations around a mean mitotic activity that is fixed at some level related to the replacement needs of that tissue. Thus, most epithelia tend to have relatively high mitotic rates, whereas most connective tissues seem to be mitotically inactive.

There are many factors that determine the mitotic rate of a tissue at a given time, including, for instance, nutritional elements and hormonal influences but the most important aspect appears to be the replacement need instigated either from within the organ, or from neuro-endocrine sources which work to maintain the body in physical balance.

TYPES OF SKIN

Except possibly in the case of identical twins, no two skins are exactly similar in type or behaviour. However, within broad limits it is possible to recognize certain characteristic types, as follows.

Soft Fair Skin

This does not pigment easily and is intolerant to ultraviolet light, thus burning easily. It is susceptible to chapping and chafing from friction, strong caustic solutions and severe cold. It is subject to reactions from epilation, and is more susceptible to eczematous reactions than the darker, pigmented skin.

Greasy Skin

This is the seborrhoeic type of skin, with an abundant secretion from the sebaceous glands of the hair follicles. It is altogether a 'tougher' skin than the fair skin, but can be prone to dandruff, seborrhoea, seborrhoeic dermatitis, acne and staphylococcal infections. There is a danger that as a result of a heat reaction in the tissues, epilation treatment will cause scarring and hyperpigmentation.

Pigmenting Skin

A dark skin and a greasy skin often occur together, and the colour is not necessarily related to that of the hair and eyes. It depends not only on the amount of melanin present, but also on the thickness of the epidermis and the degree to which the superficial blood vessels are dilated.

Common Variations of Normal Skin

XERODERMA OR DRY SKIN

This skin is dry, rough and horny on the outer surfaces of the limbs and exposed areas. It is susceptible to chapping in cold weather, and the use of soaps, detergents and antiseptics may cause eczema. Xeroderma is also associated with such allergic states as asthma, and people with this type of skin often develop a special sort of eczema—atopic eczema.

SEBORRHOEA OR GREASY SKIN

This skin is oily and the complexion muddy. The scalp is often covered with dandruff and rough, sticky looking scales. The resultant itching leads to scratching, which, in turn, often produces impetigo or boils. *Acne vulgaris* and *acne rosacea* may be present, both of which are likely to occur where there is excessive secretion of sebum from the sebaceous glands. When an eczema condition develops, it takes the special form of *seborrhoeic dermatitis* affecting the areas where hair follicles and sebaceous glands are plentiful. Individuals with seborrhoea cannot tolerate a work condition that is dirty, hot or wet, without a worsening of their skin condition.

HYPERHIDROTIC OR WET SKIN

Hyperhidrotics sweat heavily on the face, in the body flexures (folds) and on the palms of the hands and soles of the feet. This sweat washes away the protective fatty acid mantle and makes the skin more susceptible to infection—especially pyogenic or fungus infections—in these regions. Sweat dissolves substances in contact with the skin, such as dye from clothes, metal inserts in foundation garments, etc., and contact dermatitis from these causes is common. These individuals are very prone to eczema and may react badly to the trauma of the epilation process, so treatment should proceed slowly and carefully.

ANATOMY OF THE HAIR

Hairs are dead structures, composed of keratinized (horny) cells that are compactly cemented together before they leave the hair follicle cavity. They grow out of tubes of epidermal cells, which are sunk into the dermis, and receive their blood supply from capillary loops situated in the papillae of the dermal layer. Hair is a sensitive, tactile organ, and its main role now must be to increase awareness of surrounding environment through sensation and touch. It grows at an angle to the surface, so that it follows the natural contours of the body above the surface.

The hair consists of a *shaft*, the part visible above the surface, which is horny in nature, and usually pigmented. The shaft has several sections depending on the hair type: the **outer cuticle** surrounding the pigmented cells of the **cortex**, which encloses the central cells of the **medulla**. The **root** of the hair, the enclosed area or **bulb** grows from a papilla area of active cells at its lower end, and forms a column of compressed cells, which gradually harden into the shaft. The concave **dermal papilla** area derives its blood supply from the capillary loop adjacent to it, and this determines the growth and health of the hair.

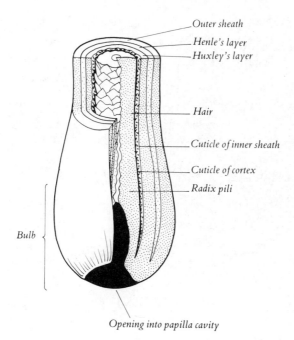

Outer sheath
Henle's layer
Huxley's layer
Hair
Cuticle of inner sheath
Cuticle of cortex
Radix pili
Bulb
Opening into papilla cavity

SECTION OF A HAIR IN A FOLLICLE

The hair **follicle** is a narrow pocket, formed partly by the dermis and partly by the epidermis. The **outer sheath** is composed of basal layer cells which follow its descent into the dermis, and the

inner sheath is formed from the horny epidermal cells. The follicle and the hair are as one, and in removal, that is, plucking, the inner sheath is visible. During its life cycle, the same hair follicle may give rise to more than one type of hair. In human skin, many of the follicles that in pre-adolescent years produce vellus-like hairs, change at puberty into large follicles that produce coarse hairs, such as on the beard. Conversely, in baldness the large follicles of the human male scalp may revert to produce lanugo-type hairs. Attached to the underside of the sloping hair follicle is a small non-striped muscle, the *arrector pili* which, under stimulus of fear, cold, etc., makes the hair stand on end.

Hair growth is continual in healthy adults, going through a cycle of growth, loss and replacement, which keeps constant the amount of hair present.

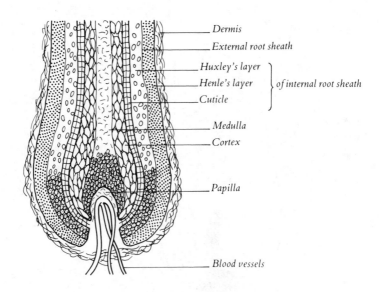

Dermis
External root sheath
Huxley's layer ⎫
Henle's layer ⎬ *of internal root sheath*
Cuticle ⎭
Medulla
Cortex
Papilla
Blood vessels

THE HAIR STRUCTURE

Structure of the Hair

CUTICLE

The cuticle is a single layer of imbricated (overlapping) cells with the free margins directed towards the tip of the hair. Although there is only one layer of cells forming the cuticle, these are so elongated that many of them overlap at any one place, making the cuticle a multi-layered structure. The scales are translucent and free of pigment. Within the follicle, the cells of the cuticle are *interlocked* with those of the inner root sheath. This arrangement firmly anchors the hair in the follicle. The cuticle of the hair binds the cortex; without this protection the cortex would become frayed and fall apart. A thin lipid and carbohydrate layer surrounds the cuticle and is thought to protect the hair from the effects of chemical and physical agents.

CORTEX

The cortex forms the bulk of the hair and is composed of elongated (fusiform), keratinized cells cemented together. In pigmented hairs, *melanin* granules are aligned longitudinally in the cells of the cortex. In the absence of pigment, hairs appear translucent. Between the cells of the cortex, variable numbers of *fusi*, delicate air spaces, are found. In the living portion of the hair root, these spaces are filled with fluid, but as the hair grows and dries out, air replaces the fluid and fusi are formed. Fusi, which are more numerous and larger in coarser hair, are bigger at the base of the hair and disappear near the tip.

MEDULLA

In the centre of the hair, we usually find a medulla, which may be continuous, discontinuous or fragmented. In the finest hairs, the medulla is most often absent; in coarse hairs, it is continuous or fragmented. The type of medulla present can vary, even within the same hair. It is composed of large, loosely connected, keratinized cells. Large intra- and inter-cellular air spaces in the medulla determine, to a great extent, the sheen and colour tones of the hair by influencing the reflection of light.

Structure of the Hair Follicle

Hair follicles are continuous with the surface epidermis by way of the **pilary canal**. They are slanted, with their roots growing down to the *panniculus adiposus*. The follicles attain their greatest diameter at their base, where they are dilated into an **onion-shaped bulb**. An obovate (egg-shaped) 'cavity' inside the bulb is completely filled with the loose connective tissue of the **dermal papilla**. The upper part of the follicle that extends from the entrance of the duct of the sebaceous glands to the surface is the pilary canal. Bundles of smooth muscle fibres, the *arrectores pilorum muscles*, extend at an acute angle from the surface of the dermis to the bulge, a swelling on the side of the follicle just below the level of the sebaceous glands. These muscles, stimulated (innervated) largely by adrenergic nerves, contract under stress, pull the hair to a vertical position and draw the skin around the follicles, giving rise to the elevation known as 'goose flesh' or *cutis anserina*. Vellus hair follicles have no arrectores pilorum muscles.

Hair follicles are composed of an **outer root sheath**, an **inner root sheath** and the **hair** in the centre. The thickness of the outer sheath is proportional to the size of the hair follicle, and is thick in the follicles of large hairs. The inner root sheath is composed of three concentric layers: *Henle's layer* on the outside is one cell thick and rests against the outer root sheath; *Huxley's layer* in the middle is two or more cells thick; and the *single-layered cuticle* of the inner sheath on the inside rests against the hair. The cuticle of the inner sheath is a layer of imbricated, scale-like, keratinized cells, the free borders of which are directed to, and interlock with, the cuticle cells of the hair.

Hair follicles are surrounded by a **connective tissue sheath** in which the fibres of the inner layer are arranged circularly, and those of the outer layer are disposed longitudinally. The outer root sheath is separated from the connective tissue sheath by a hyalin, non-cellular, glassy or **vitreous membrane**. The connective tissue sheath is continuous above with the papillary body of the dermis, and with the **dermal papilla** at the base of the follicle. Since these three connective tissue structures are continuous, they can be considered as a united tissue structure. The hair follicle, then, is not in contact with the fibrous reticular layer of the dermis.

BULB

The bulb of the hair follicle can be divided into a lower region of undifferentiated (undetermined) cells and an upper region in which the cells become differentiated to form the inner sheath and the hair. A line across the widest part of the papilla would separate the two regions at the **'critical' level**. Below the critical level is the **matrix**, or germination centre of the follicle, where every cell is mitotically active. From the matrix, cells move to the upper part of the bulb, where they increase in volume and become elongated vertically. Some of the cells in the upper bulb still show some signs of mitotic activity, but these are too few to account for much of the growth of the hair.

In the topmost part of the bulb, in the keratogenous zone, the cells become hyalinized and the keratin of the hair is stabilized. Depending upon the length of the follicle, the **keratogenous zone** ends at approximately one-third of the way between the tip of the papilla and the surface of the skin.

Melanin in the follicle is distributed in a remarkably rigid pattern. Since the matrix has almost no melanin, the separation of the upper from the lower bulb at the critical level is remarkably clear. The outer and inner sheaths are free of melanin. Traces of pigment may occasionally spill into the inner sheath and very small dendritic cells are found there on rare occasions, but the dividing line is very sharp between the cells of the hair itself, which are pigmented, and those of the sheaths, which are not. Most of the tall, columnar cells lining the dermal papilla are melanin-producing dendritic melanocytes. The dendrites that radiate from these cells are insinuated between the undifferentiated cells of the medulla and the cortex. As the cells of the hair cortex move up from the matrix, they acquire pigment granules. The upper bulb is comparable to the spinous layer of the epidermis. In both places, epidermal cells become larger, acquire pigment, synthesize fibrous proteins, become reorientated, and undergo the final steps of keratinization.

INNER ROOT SHEATH

The inner root sheath of active hair follicles consists of Henle's and Huxley's layers and the cuticle. All three layers arise from the cells of the matrix. The cells move upwards and laterally (outwards) from the matrix and become arranged into three concentric layers in the upper bulb. In the upper region of the bulb, the cells of Henle's layer become hyalinized. About midway up the follicle, the cells of Huxley's layer become hyalinized. Shortly after this, the cuticle cells also become hyalinized, and above the middle of the follicle all three layers become fused. It is at the halfway level of the follicle that the cells of the cuticle become slightly dislocated axially (sideways) with the free margins directed downwards, so becoming interlocked with the cells of the cuticle of the hair.

The inner sheath is eliminated in the philosebaceous canal, probably as a result of a chemical change (the enzyme keratinase may digest it), but the hair shaft, being slightly more acidic and covered by a film of lipids and carbohydrates, would be protected from enzymatic action.

OUTER ROOT SHEATH

The thickness of the outer sheath is uneven, causing the hair to be eccentric (off centre) in the follicle. Most of the follicles have some degree of swelling of the outer sheath on the side of the bulge. At the level of the sebaceous glands, and above, the outer sheath is indistinguishable from the surface epidermis.

The outer sheath extends all the way up to the tip of the bulb; at that point, it is composed of two layers of greatly flattened cells. Just above the bulb, the outer sheath develops three layers and attains its greatest thickness about a third of the way up the follicle. About halfway up the follicle, the cytoplasm of the cells that rest against Henle's layer becomes hyalinized and undergoes partial keratinization. Some mitotic activity is found in the upper part of the follicle where the outer sheath blends with the surface epidermis. This part is similar to the surface epidermis, and forms a keratinized surface layer which is constantly being sloughed (cast) off. Lower down in the follicle, the outer sheath is a morphologically static structure—that is, its form does not change.

VITREOUS MEMBRANE

The vitreous membrane is a non-cellular partition that separates the outer root sheath from the connective tissue sheath. It varies in thickness over the length of the follicle: thickest around the widest part of the bulb. It is very thin around the lower part of the bulb, and seems to be non-existent in the papilla cavity.

The membrane is composed of two layers: the outer layer surrounds the entire follicle and is continuous with the basement membrane of the epidermis. The second, inner layer is found in the lower half of the hair follicle.

CONNECTIVE TISSUE SHEATH

The connective tissue sheath is composed of an inner layer with fibres arranged circularly and a thicker outer layer with longitudinal fibres. Both layers are composed of collagenous fibres, a few elastic fibres and fibroblasts; neither layer abounds in cells, but more may be found in the outer one. The blood vessels of the follicle are embedded in the connective tissue sheath. Plexuses of capillaries are found mostly in the inner layer, while the straight parallel arterioles are round in the outer layer. The connective tissue sheath is continuous with both the thin layer of areolar tissue and the papillary layer of the dermis. At the base of the dermis, the connection tissue sheath is attached to the dermal papilla by a stalk. Thus, the connective tissue sheath, the papillary layer of the dermis and the dermal papilla comprise a continuous unit of tissue.

DERMAL PAPILLA

The term 'dermal papilla' should be used to designate only the *connective tissue* element which is enclosed by the bulb of the hair follicle during anagen and which forms a compact ball of dermal cells underneath the 'hair germ' during telogen. The dermal papilla is attached to the connective tissue sheath by a stalk. It is richly vascularized in large hair follicles, less so in smaller ones and not at all in the follicles of lanugo hairs. The papilla is pointed at its summit. In the follicles of *pili multigemini* (multiple hairs), the papilla is split into two or three more parts, ranging from one papilla with two apices (tips) to completely separate papillae.

THE HAIR GROWTH CYCLE

The Biology of Hair Growth

When a follicle ceases to produce a hair, it shrivels up and the lower part or bulb largely degenerates, its role fulfilled for the time being. These resting or quiescent follicles are simpler in structure and much shorter than active ones. At the base of a resting follicle the hair, if still present, forms a *club* that is anchored by thin keratinous strands to the surrounding epithelial sac. The club is surrounded by a hyaline capsule, the remnants of the inner root sheath: which continues up to just below the duct of the sebaceous gland, where it becomes wrinkled and fragmented. Around the capsule, the remaining outer root sheath forms a thickened epithelial sac at the base of which is a peg of cells. Below the flattened base of this peg of cells is the ball of *dermal papilla* cells, which are no longer encapsulated by a bulb. Close inspection of a hair epilated during the resting stage will show that it sits in a very shallow position, almost on the skin's surface, and has a blob-like dot or full stop on its root end. This rounded club is called the *pedicle of cells* and the lower part of the epithelial sac called the *hair germ*, and it is from this hair germ that the next generation of hairs develops.

Changes in the body can swiftly affect the hair growth pattern, either increasing its renewal rate or decreasing its capacity to regenerate correctly. Endocrine influence on the hair follicles can result in unwanted hair in women, and is responsible for male baldness. The hair follicle responds to the messages it receives from the endocrine system, and its pattern of growth is altered accordingly. Healthy hair growth in the young person may be found to have few resting follicles, with hairs being replaced before the old club hair is shed naturally. These double-haired follicles are simply skipping the resting stage, and the old club hair and the new finely pointed hair can be observed emerging from the same follicle. So the new hair is established before the old one is lost.

This growth pattern can be stated very simply in the following way:

(1) Growing hairs are said to be in **anagen**.
(2) Resting or quiescent follicles are said to be in **telogen**.
(3) Transitionary follicles in the stage between anagen and telogen are said to be in **catagen**.

So the sequence of events, if simplified, becomes anagen–catagen–telogen and is repeated constantly until a hair ceases to be formed due to internal influences. It is important to remember that very few external influences have any effect on hair growth, apart from disease of the actual follicle structure. The strength, vitality, colour and texture of the hair are determined from within. Certain treatments such as plucking or waxing are thought to increase the growth of hair follicles, but this is due to the disruption in the growth cycle rather than any actual increase in growth. If all the hairs in an area were to be removed at the same time, as is done with waxing,

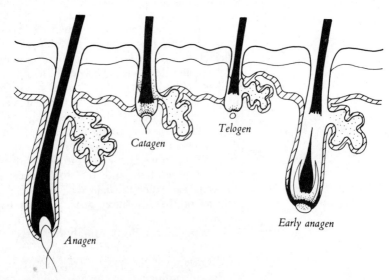

Catagen

Telogen

Anagen

Early anagen

DIFFERENT STAGES OF HAIR GROWTH

it would be seen that there are hairs present in all the various stages of growth: some resting, some in catagen and many growing in the anagen stage. By inspecting the wax strip after removal of hairs, it is easy to determine the different stages of growth, due to obvious differences in length and structure of the hairs present. However, although all the hairs were at different stages when they were removed, they will all begin regrowth from the same stage after the follicles have recovered. In fact, waxing acts to bring the hair follicles into a regularized pattern of growth which would not be found naturally.

How hairs react to this disruption in their natural cycle gives rise to the widely differing views held about the reaction of waxing and other methods of non-permanent hair removal on the overall pattern of growth. In some cases, the hair appears to grow more quickly and more thickly and in others to have slowed down and be sparser in character. Insufficient study has been completed to be able to form definite statements regarding alterations in the growth patterns. Experience has shown, however, that general health, age and hormone influences have the greatest effect on the hair growth overall. Into the same category of undiscovered knowledge comes the question as to why hairs turn white and why only some men become bald prematurely. If an external application for increasing hair growth did exist, bald men would have used it long ago.

THE RESTING HAIR FOLLICLE
TELOGEN

In considering the simplest of the stages of the growth cycle first, it is necessary to understand the structure of the follicle, so that the following more active stages can be understood. In a resting follicle, two physiologically distinct regions are apparent: one above the level of the duct of the sebaceous gland, and the other one below. In the *upper region*, the cells of which are in direct continuity with the surface epidermis, the mitotic activity of the basal cell layer is similar to that of the basal layer of the epidermis, but in the *lower region* the cells are mitotically inert. In the upper follicle, there is an open space or channel between the follicle wall and the hair shaft. In the lower follicle, the walls press closely on to the hair, which at its base has a strong brush-like attachment to the surrounding cell mass. Beneath the follicle base is the small dermal papilla.

The follicle appears collapsed, like an empty stocking: deflated, waiting for the leg to refill it.

Telogen

The follicle may stay in this state for some considerable length of time. Hair does appear to grow less at certain times of the year and whether or not this is due to dietary influences seems uncertain.

EARLY FOLLICLE GROWTH ANAGEN STAGE 1

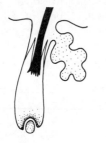

Early anagen
stage I

The first sign of that mitotic activity which results in the production of a new hair is seen in the basal cells of the lower follicle—these cells grow downwards as a solid column of undifferentiated and dividing cells to surround the dermal papilla. Then, the lower part of the follicle starts to grow downwards, with the role of many of its cells as yet undetermined. There is no mitotic activity in that part of the lower follicle which surrounds the brush or club-like base of the old hair, while in the upper follicle regular mitotic activity continues as normal.

LATER FOLLICLE GROWTH ANAGEN STAGES II AND III

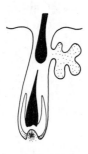

Later follicle growth
Anagen stage II

As the new follicle elongates rapidly, the inner follicle sheath and the tip of the newly forming hair begin to differentiate, and the cells involved cease to show mitosis. From the base upwards, the sequence is as follows:

(1) The basal region of very increased mitotic activity takes the form of a ring which surrounds the dermal papilla.

(2) Next, a narrow region of differentiation appears, where no mitosis is seen. The cells are becoming organized, but in this section they are not involved with growing.

(3) Then, a rapidly elongating region appears, containing in the centre the newly differentiating hair, and peripherally (around the outer perimeter) a zone of active mitosis in which many of the new cells involved in the lengthening of the hair follicle are produced. Until the follicle is fully grown, the lengthening of the follicle keeps exact pace with the lengthening of the new hair shaft. Consequently, the hair tip always remains the same distance beneath the brush-like club attachment of the old hair.

(4) The non-mitotic zone surrounding the brush-like club attachment of the old hair remains unchanged.

(5) The cells of the upper follicle now show an increased rate of mitosis, and a similar increase in the mitotic activity takes place in the overlying surface epidermis.

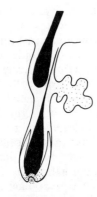

Anagen stage III

THE FULLY GROWN FOLLICLE
ANAGEN STAGES IV AND V

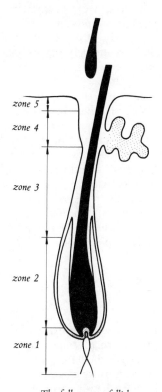

zone 5

zone 4

zone 3

zone 2

zone 1

The fully grown follicle
Anagen stage IV and V

When its growth is complete, the follicle is at least six times longer than it was in the resting stage. From the base upwards, the sequence of zones is as follows:

(1) The cells of the basal, ring-like matrix show violent mitotic activity which, however, ceases abruptly at a point level with the tip of the dermal papilla.

(2) Above the dermal papilla is a zone in which the cells arrange themselves into columns, and in which they begin to elongate and differentiate. No mitotic activity is present.

(3) Above this is the keratogenous zone in which the cells are keratinized to form a recognizable hair. They lose moisture and harden. No mitotic activity (cellular division) is seen in any of these cells, or in the cells of the surrounding follicle wall.

(4) With the point of the new hair now forcing upwards the brush-like attachment of the old hair and the surrounding cells are pushed to one side. These surrounding cells show no mitotic activity and are subsequently shed.

(5) The cells of the upper follicle show a subnormal mitotic rate, and a similar subnormal mitotic rate is found in the overlying epidermis. The growing process is now over for the time being and the surface skin returns to a near-normal state.

THE FINAL STAGE CATAGEN

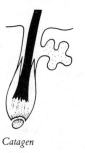

Catagen

When the new hair is fully grown, mitotic activity in the basal, ring-like cell matrix suddenly ceases, and the new hair develops a brush-like attachment to the cell mass which surrounds its base. The work of the follicle in developing a new hair is now largely completed and, its usefulness temporarily over, its structure changes again. There follows the rapid degeneration and destruction of a greater part of the lower follicle. The outer root sheath in the upper part of a follicle forms at least part of the 'hair germ' and the epidermal sac around the club hair. The inner layers of the vitreous membrane become extremely thick and form a wrinkled sac around the degenerating lower part of the follicle. (In telogen this becomes fragmented and is reabsorbed.) Resting hair follicles are surrounded by only a thin hyaline membrane which corresponds to the outer layer of the vitreous membrane. The connective tissue sheath becomes wrinkled and thickened. (In quiescent follicles, the connective tissue sheath becomes fragmented and is reabsorbed, leaving only a wispy trail in the area vacated by the follicle.) So the process has come full cycle, and by this complex, yet orderly process the follicle returns to its normal resting length, its task of producing a new replacement hair over for the time being.

The fact that hairs have a predetermined cycle is obvious from the length that hairs attain in different parts of the body—eye lashes, arm and leg hairs having different length potential to hair on the head. Only individuals with a prolonged growth cycle, for example, could grow their hair to below the waist, and many people can never achieve more than shoulder-length hair. At an average growth rate of half an inch a month, waist-length hair is obviously several years old and must have a very spaced-out replacement growth cycle.

EMBRYOLOGY OF HAIR— HOW A FOLLICLE AND HAIR FORMS IN THE UNBORN CHILD

The follicle and its hair must always be considered as one, in its *formation*, *growth* and *renewal*—it is often referred to as the *philo-sebaceous unit*. Nowhere can this be seen more clearly than when the forming follicle and its hair is considered in the human foetus.

First the hair follicle is developed from epithelial cells which quickly become organized into recognizable areas of the fully formed hair follicle, able to be distinguished as distinct components making up the philo-sebaceous unit. This changing process is known as differentiation.

Differentiation

This differentiation can best be described as a process where cells grow or become different in the process of growth and development. The cells of the follicle and its hair have, like all cells of the body, to follow this process, and full formation is achieved in a very ordered and predictable manner.

At a very early stage in the follicle's development, differentiation occurs, and even though in an embryo stage, distinct parts of the future follicle can be distinguished. The cells have a growth pattern to follow in their development, and this can be looked at closely to see differentiation in process in the forming follicle and its hair.

Differentiation also occurs in the renewal process of the fully formed follicle, when one hair is shed (catagen and telogen) and replaced by another newly formed hair (anagen). As the follicle regenerates and grows its new hair to replace the lost hair, its cells quickly gain their future identity. This is most clearly seen as the forming hair shaft passes through the critical level and becomes hard and keratinized rather than soft and pliable. The cells have taken on their permanent role as a recognizable hair.

So differentiation is a growth and change process involved in the forming follicle and hair, and its renewal process in normal life, when fully formed.

Pre-germ—Primitive Hair Germ Stage

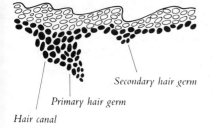

Secondary hair germ

Primary hair germ

Hair canal

In the unborn child where a follicle will form, a crowding of nuclei occurs in the basal layer of the epidermis, and this is known as the *primitive hair germ* or *pre-germ stage*. At this stage the epidermis often consists of only two layers, germinal cells and periderm, but development of a third intermediate layer may be present. The nuclei of the stratum germinativum and intermedium become more numerous and are smaller. It is considered that initially neighbouring cells are drawn into forming the hair germ (*invagination*) while later the follicle grows by mitotic (cellular) division of its own cells.

The Hair Germ Stage

The pre-germ rapidly becomes the hair germ, and the nuclei become longer, elongated downwards into the corium of the skin. Additional cells accumulate above the basal layer, beneath the periderm. As the hair germ develops it assumes the slant of the fully formed hair angle, growing obliquely downwards.

In young embryos the entire epidermis including the basal layer is laden with glycogen. In the forming hair germs cells this substance is lost

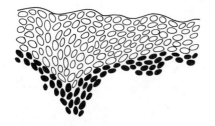

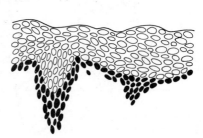

progressively, and a dividing membrane (basement membrane) becomes evident. At this stage an accumulation of mesodermal nuclei is obvious around the bulge of the basal layer.

Hair Peg Stage

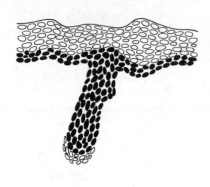

The outer cells of the hair peg are arranged radially around the long central axis or core, like a column. Cells in the centre of the core initially have no direction, but quickly become arranged longitudinally to form the central column. The most active area is the broadest advancing part of the peg, destined to become the *matrix*. The broad end may be flat at its base or slightly concave due to pressure against the compacted ball of mesodermal cells—the future *dermal papilla*. The entire column is enclosed in a sheath of mesodermal cells, continuous with those of the papilla. As the young follicle becomes elongated, first its central cells and later the outer border (peripheral) basal cells begin to acquire glycogen again, with the exception of the tall matrix cells which always remain free of it.

Beginning of Differentiation —Bulbous Peg Stage

As the follicle lengthens, differentiation of its parts begins. The advancing border enlarges, becomes bulbous and envelops part of the mesodermal material which is divided into the egg-shaped papilla inside the hollowed-out bulb of the matrix, and the papillary pad below the bulb. Papilla and pad are connected by a gradually narrowing neck.

At the same time two solid epithelial swellings develop at the side of the follicle column. The lower swelling (known as the bulge) remains solid and its cells grow rich in glycogen, as does the rest of the follicle. Inconspicuous in adult life, this bulge is very evident in embryonic life. The

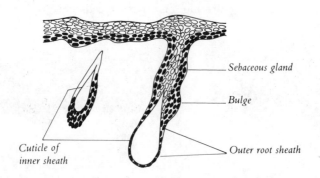

Sebaceous gland

Bulge

Cuticle of inner sheath

Outer root sheath

swelling which will become the sebaceous gland is free of glycogen at this stage. A solid cord of elongated cells extends backwards within the epidermis, and represents the hair canal.

Now the last constant part of the pilary unit begins to form, being the arrector pili muscle, which draws the adult follicle upright forming 'goose pimples' on the skin's surface. A little way from the sebaceous gland, mesodermal cells arrange themselves in a slender row, parallel to the follicle, and the arrector pili muscle is formed. It gradually extends backwards towards the 'bulge'. Up to this stage the follicle is a solid epithelial structure surrounded by a mesodermal sheath.

Differentiation of Various Parts

When all components of the philo-sebaceous follicle are apparent, growth and differentiation continue in a regulated pattern until the fully formed follicle is present. Several areas of the follicle can be recognized at this stage:

The bulb—comprising the matrix of the hair and its sheaths and mesodermal papilla.

The lower follicle—from the upper end of the bulb to the area of the bulge.

The bulge area.

The isthmus—an area between the bulge and the sebaceous gland.

The sebaceous gland area.

The infundibulum—which is the term used for the area from the point of entry of the sebaceous gland into the follicle, to the base of the epidermis. The infundibulum also continues within the epidermis as the hair canal.

The hair canal.

All these areas eventually are traversed or crossed by the *hair and inner root sheath*. In addition the arrector pili muscle and the sweat glands must be considered.

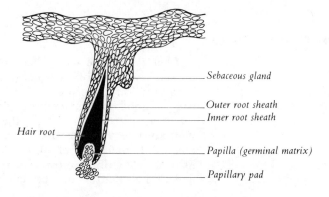

Sebaceous gland

Outer root sheath
Inner root sheath

Hair root

Papilla (germinal matrix)

Papillary pad

Early Stages of Follicle Growth and Hair Formation

The lower bulbous end of the follicle harbours the *mesodermal papilla* which consists of closely packed cells. Scattered granules of glycogen often are present in the cells of the papilla, with even more in the sub-papillary pad. As the follicle lengthens rapidly, the inner follicle sheath and the tip of the newly forming hair begin to differentiate. The most active area of cellular growth is around the papillary pad, the matrix area and, inside the concave cavity housing, the mesodermal papilla (dermal papilla).

Around the outer perimeter of the hair core there is also a zone of active mitosis in which are produced many of the new cells involved in the lengthening of the follicle, keeping exact pace with the lengthening of the new hair shaft.

So the follicle grows downwards from its base, and peripherally as well, from a rapidly elongated region approximately a third of the way up the follicle's total length from its base.

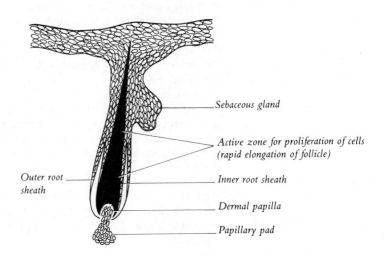

Sebaceous gland

Active zone for proliferation of cells (rapid elongation of follicle)

Outer root sheath

Inner root sheath

Dermal papilla

Papillary pad

Fully Formed Follicle

When the follicle and its hair are fully formed, the activity of the follicle alters as its role changes. From now on its purpose will be to maintain the hair in good health, and respond to messages received internally through the bloodstream, which dictate when the hair will be shed, and need renewal. In the course of normal life, hair changes its form many times, most of these changes being under the control of the endocrine system, through hormonal influences. The follicle will respond to these stimuli by shedding hairs, growing new hairs in the original or an altered form, or simply growing the existing hair in a stronger or more frail version.

So it can be seen how lanugo hair becomes normal soft vellus hair, and how normal hair can become coarse sexual hair at puberty. It also shows how a follicle normally producing a fine vellus hair, can be instigated into growing an unwanted disfiguring superflous hair, simply because it responds to hormonal messages received through the blood vessels meshing around the follicle.

So the follicle and its hair (philo-sebaceous unit) are very adaptable in life. This flexibility is achieved by maintaining the unit in normal health, and having the capacity for changes, built into its development (see The Hair Growth Cycle).

The fully formed follicle maintains its health and the growth of the hair protruding from the skin's surface in several ways. The matrix area of the follicle remains active to continue the growth of the actual hair itself. The activity ceases at the hair's 'critical' level, a point level with the tip of the dermal papilla area. Further up the follicle the cells organize themselves into columns, elongate and differentiate, and acquire pigment molecules. They also become keratinized and start to form a hair, losing moisture and become hard, forming

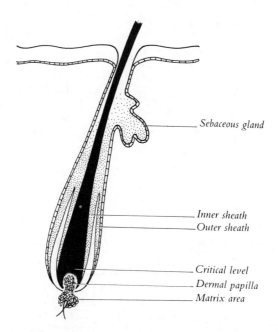

Sebaceous gland

Inner sheath
Outer sheath

Critical level
Dermal papilla
Matrix area

the shaft of the hair as it emerges from the skin. The upper follicle and epidermal areas also show a subnormal mitotic rate, and the sebaceous gland through its secretion (sebum) lubricates the shaft of the hair and helps keep it in good health.

So only the base of the follicle is active at this maintenance stage and awaits further instruction about future patterns of growth.

Chapter 4

Consultation Techniques and Treatment Organization

From the very first application of electrology on a client, even within the training situation, it is important to consider *client handling* as an essential part of technique. Considerate handling and a sympathetic approach will improve a client's capacity for treatment by reducing discomfort and nervous tension.

The initial consultation is a very important part of the client handling procedure, not only in providing the necessary information to plan and carry out the treatment programme, but also, and quite as important, in establishing a good relationship between electrologist and client. This is essential if the ensuing treatment is to be completely successful. Also, in professional practice, the initial consultation has commercial relevance, for its success can determine whether a client is gained or not. In addition, as many operators work for themselves, running their own businesses, gaining new clients and retaining their regular clientele is obviously essential. Consultation procedures, therefore, are vital in achieving business and professional success and must be learned alongside other practical abilities and theoretical knowledge.

THE CONSULTATION

When a client comes for a consultation regarding the possibility of undergoing epilation treatment, she may be very apprehensive and will need to be put at her ease. The electrologist must seek to reduce the client's nervous tension while, at the same time, promoting confidence in her ability to provide a solution to the problem. The initial consultation may be of only a few minutes' duration and possibly linked with a short introductory treatment, so that the client can actually experience what is being discussed. However, what is said in these few minutes will almost certainly decide whether or not you have gained a new client.

Appearance

Personal appearance is the most immediate factor in determining the successful outcome of this initial consultation. It must inspire confidence. A clean, white clinical-style overall should be worn as this helps to establish the professional standard of work that the client can expect. Badges of professional associations, which denote the level of training received, should be worn with pride. These inspire tremendous confidence, and instil in the client the feeling that she is in the hands of an expert, trained to solve her hair problems. The electrologist should have tidy hair and short, well-kept nails, both to create a good impression and to allow hygienic and efficient work. Nothing would be more off-putting to a potential client than an operator with a slovenly manner, unkempt hair and painted, claw-like nails.

So much is judged from this first appearance that students should train themselves always to be immaculately turned out, so that it becomes automatic and a routine part of their professional life.

Client Handling Ability

It is important that the client is put sufficiently at ease to allow her to ask any questions regarding the treatment which may be bothering her. Discussion should take place concerning the way in which the treatment would be organized specifically to suit the client's particular hair condition, and also ways of maintaining an appearance during the period of treatment which would not be embarrassing to her. The client must be made to feel that not only is a solution possible, but that this is the ideal person to achieve it. The electrologist must develop the ability to sell herself, for the client has the power of choice.

Knowledge

Having both a complete knowledge of the subject and the ability to impart some of that knowledge to the client builds confidence on both sides. Commonsense will guide the electrologist as to the amount of detail required in explaining the treatment. In many cases, the client will feel fully confident in the operator's qualifications and will be happy to leave the entire matter in her hands, not wishing to know anything about the technique. In other cases, in order to avoid misunderstanding about such things as length of treatment time, regrowth, etc., it will be necessary to explain briefly the epilation procedure, how it works, its limitations and so on. In all cases, clients must have sufficient understanding of the procedure to co-operate with aspects of treatment organization such as regular attendance and home-care measures to ensure success and avoid skin damage.

Every consultation will be different, depending on the client's hair condition and also on her prior knowledge about permanent hair removal. The client may have received an explanatory leaflet about epilation from the clinic in response to a telephone or written enquiry, and this will have answered many of her questions. She may also have read magazine features about the technique, and felt it could be the answer to her problem. The client may understand permanent removal to be 'electrolysis', which, as we have seen, though not strictly correct, acts as a useful umbrella title for all permanent removal, being so well established in the public's mind. There is no need for lengthy explanations. Generally speaking, the client is interested in results not the means by which they are accomplished. A brief and simplified explanation of the technique and treatment organization are the basic elements which need to be got across to the client.

Checklist of Important Points

It is useful in the early days, when gaining experience, to have a list of points to be covered briefly in the initial interview. This helps to ensure that the electrologist puts the client fully in the picture, answers questions she may not have thought of or was too embarrassed to ask, and still leaves time for questions without making the consultation time too long. It is vital to gain the client's co-operation regarding regular attendance, home-care, etc., in order to achieve a successful result. This is far more likely to occur if she has a good understanding of the technique and the procedures necessary.

The points to be covered in the consultation are outlined below:

(1) Inspection of the face or treatment area and discussion of hair growth.
(2) Discussion of temporary methods of hair removal previously used.
(3) Emphasis on the permanence of epilation (or electrolysis if the client recognizes the process by this title).
(4) Explanation of the epilation process, with emphasis on epilation as the only *permanent* solution.
(5) Description of the hair and follicle and the hair destruction process, and discussion of the relationship of regrowth hair.

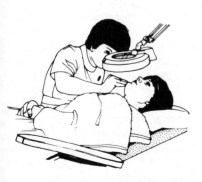

CLIENT AND ELECTROLOGIST
IN CONSULTATION SITUATION

(6) Explanation of treatment procedures, length of appointments, time between treatments.
(7) Discussion of cost of treatment.
(8) Confirmation that, with a skilled, qualified operator, no skin damage or marking will result.
(9) Explanation of difficulty of prognosis regarding hair growth, skin sensitivity and overall progress.

The client may ask questions at any stage of the consultation and these can be answered briefly. If the client has undergone professional treatment previously she will probably already understand the procedure, in which case it will only be necessary to record her personal details on her record card. The electrologist should feel that at the end of the consultation the client understands all the above points, either from prior knowledge, or as a result of the consultation. As time is money to the operator, each consultation must be justified in terms of the additional work it provides for her. Consultations are normally completely free, or charged as a short-duration appointment if practical treatment is combined with the consultation.

The checklist is also useful as a reminder to the practising electrologist of points to cover in the consultation, so as to prevent the client from going away from the 'initial visit' without essential information relevant to treatment success.

These points will now be considered in more detail for reference.

INSPECTION OF THE FACE OR TREATMENT AREA

After a few words of greeting and explanation, the prospective client should be seated in a clinic chair and the hair growth and skin condition inspected and discussed. The strength of the hair growth, how quickly it returns after temporary removal, its position and character must all be considered in assessing the growth condition and likely pattern of improvement. The client must be informed about the possibility of hairs emerging during the early stages of treatment as a result of previous hair removal methods such as plucking and waxing. In addition, skin marking, scars, skin eruptions and general skin sensitivity should all be noticed and recorded. The role of hormonal imbalance in relation to the client's hair growth condition should be considered; the client's age and circumstances have tremendous relevance here, and the possibility of medical referral must be borne in mind.

TEMPORARY METHODS OF HAIR REMOVAL USED

It should be explained that the way in which hairs have previously been removed—whether by plucking, waxing, cutting, shaving or using depilatory creams—has a direct bearing on the progress that can be expected and the fact that all these methods are temporary and the hairs will always return should be stressed, so that the permanence of epilation can be seen as a beneficial alternative. The client should be informed that previous waxing and plucking of the hairs may have caused distortion of the follicles, thus making probing difficult and regrowth more persistent. It is important not to depress the client about this point, but simply to present it as a fact to be overcome and as explanation for the increased level of regrowth which will be forthcoming initially. Methods of temporary removal that are permissible during treatment should be discussed and how these can be accomplished so as not to slow down or interfere with the epilation progress. The sensitizing effect of depilatory creams on skin tissues should be mentioned and discussed in more detail with the client who prefers this method of hair removal. It should be noted that as depilatory creams work by dissolving keratinized horny tissue, they act on skin tissue as well as hair structures, so leaving the skin rather exposed, sensitive and easily irritated, and the client should be advised that, as this can bring about increased skin reaction to epilation and slow healing, this method of temporary hair removal should not be used during the treatment programme, and cutting or shaving suggested as alternatives.

PERMANENCE OF THE EPILATION METHOD

The eventual *permanence* of epilation should be stressed, although it appears a long, tedious and exacting treatment. It should be explained that each hair has to be treated individually, which makes the treatment a lengthy business, but that once a follicle's capacity to grow a hair is destroyed, it can never produce a new hair. So, although the follicle may need several treatments to accomplish destruction if the growth is strong, once completed, *no more hairs can grow*. The ultimate aim, a hair-free appearance, should be stressed in discussion, and the client urged to think of each hair treated as one hair less and thus a reduction of the problem and embarrassment. The client should be encouraged to understand that epilation is a permanent solution, although one that seems far off in the future and that the permanency lies in the individual treatment of each hair, and in this way gain some acceptance of the long-term nature of the treatment programme.

EXPLANATION OF THE EPILATION PROCESS

The method by which epilation destroys the hair can best be described to the client as electrical heat which cauterizes the hair root by using a special kind of current which does not cause shocks or harm to the individual, but is capable of completely destroying the hair without skin injury, if skilfully applied. This alerts the client as to the sensation that will be experienced, which can be pictured as a hot or sharp prick, lasting only a fraction of a second. It is best to avoid using the terms 'burning sensations' or 'burning the root', as these suggest a far worse sensation than most clients experience, and, the power of suggestion being strong, the client may suffer far more discomfort than she need. With the latest epilation machines discomfort is much reduced, a result of intensive development from manufacturers to improve this aspect of treatment, whilst maintaining effective results.

DESCRIPTION OF THE HAIR AND FOLLICLE

It is useful to describe to the client the structure of the hair and follicle, in order to show the need for careful, skilled work. Often a wall chart or diagram of the hair helps here, and in many cases it may not even be necessary to involve the client to this extent. A diagram of the hair and follicle structure does provide an instant means of demonstrating why regrowth can occur, or why follicle distortion from previous interference does cause treatment problems. The areas of active growth can be shown and discussed in relation to accuracy of work. Some clients are very interested in the background to their hair condition, others not at all, so electrologists should use their own judgement in this matter.

THE HAIR DESTRUCTION PROCESS

Explain how the needle is inserted painlessly down the follicle, and how the electrical current flows through to the tip of the needle to produce a cautery in the active area of the follicle, thus coagulating the tissues, freeing the hair, and reducing or stopping the follicle's capacity to grow a new hair. Stress that it is not so much the existing hair that is being destroyed but rather the follicle's capacity to grow new hairs, that when the active area at the base of the follicle is incapable of producing more cells, *then hair cannot grow from that follicle.* Although this explanation must be simple, it is important, for it not only demonstrates the permanence of epilation, but also prepares the client for the fact that results will be *eventual*, not instantaneous. If she understands the need for care and accuracy in treatment, she will not be too impatient for results, and will appreciate why regrowth can occur.

TREATMENT PROCEDURES

Organization of the treatment programme should be discussed; the electrologist should suggest how the results can best be obtained, and should specify the duration of the appointments and how far apart they must be spaced in order to allow the skin to heal properly, especially for work centred on just one area such as the upper lip. Appointments or sittings can vary in length— ten to fifteen minutes, twenty minutes, half an hour, or even an hour or two in the case of leg hair removals—depending on the strength of the growth, the skin's sensitivity and the client's capacity for the treatment. If the client has a widespread problem such as lip, chin *and* throat hair growth, areas can be worked in rotation, and only the client's finances and the time she has available limit how much work can be done.

Leg hair and body epilation also are similar in this respect, in that it is not the skin that restricts the work, rather the time and money the client can afford to spend. The electrologist must *always* be the one who determines the length and spacing of the treatments, not the client, who naturally enough wants results as quickly as possible, and will often do anything to be rid of her hairs.

If the hair problem is severe, then it can be stressed that, initially, the more treatment time the client can give, the faster results can be seen. Obviously, this is only possible if the skin condition can stand it and the client has a good tolerance to the treatment. No *one* area can be worked on with less then ten to fourteen days between treatments, but if *many* areas are under treatment, the normal fifteen minute appointment will not go far towards solving the problem.

COST OF TREATMENT

The individual cost of *each* treatment should be stated and reference made to the fact that it is an on-going and long-term form of treatment. This gives the client an opportunity to budget for her treatments and make regular provision for them in her income. It is better not to try to give any indication as to the overall length or cost of the treatment programme, because, apart from being a depressing factor, it is often quite impossible to tell initially how long a condition may take to resolve. Like many other grooming treatments, clients get used to budgeting for their epilation, and class it together with foot care, hair care, etc., as necessary parts of life.

SKILLED OPERATOR

Clients may be apprehensive about the outcome of the treatment and concerned about the risks of scarring and skin damage, but they may be too embarrassed to bring this up themselves, so it is better if this point is introduced by the operator during the consultation while explaining the effects of the treatment. It can be simply stated that a skilled operator will cause no skin marking, although a slight redness will appear after each treatment, which will soon disappear. In some cases, the skin may react initially to epilation, but the treatment can be adjusted to suit the skin condition and in time it will revert to normal. Even a skilled operator cannot always tell exactly what reaction to expect, and so she works carefully until this knowledge is gained.

The client will gain confidence regarding treatment if she feels the operator is well-qualified and experienced. A display of diplomas in the working clinic or reception area quietly state the level of qualification, and evidence of a well-run, busy practice is additional proof of the operator's ability and experience. All this combines to tell the client she is in good hands; this is of tremendous psychological importance, and helps to ensure the success of the treatment.

DIFFICULTY OF PROGNOSIS

The client will want to know how severe a problem she has in terms of the treatment needed, and how quickly it can be resolved. It should be explained that it is difficult to assess accurately how long the treatment will last for several reasons:

(1) the strength and stubbornness of the growth;
(2) the sensitivity of the skin—severe reaction acting as a limitation;
(3) the ability of the client and her skin to stand high current intensity;
(4) the response to treatment, which is more rapid in some cases than others;
(5) the need for a conscientious approach to treatment by the client—regular appointments, home-care, etc.

If the condition is severe, and therefore the period of treatment inevitably lengthy, then it is tactful to stress that the client can look forward to the rest of her life free from her hair problem once the condition is resolved. This will help her to view the time required for treatment as short compared to the years of misery and embarrassment which she might suffer if she remained untreated. Emphasis should be placed on the improvement in appearance that each treatment brings.

Practical Epilation

The next stage is to actually apply the epilation treatment, in a modified form, so that the client can experience the sensation and adjust to it. If the client has never had epilation in any form previously, one or two probes can be applied on the less sensitive areas of the arms or legs, and then treatment progressed to the facial area. Probes should be applied slowly, with pauses between each one, using only a low current strength initially, until the client gets used to the pricking sensation and settles down. In any event, the first introductory treatment should be kept short. The client is bound to be suffering from a certain amount of nervous tension on the first visit and this may cause her to feel more discomfort than usual. This could result in a headache after treatment; this is due purely to tension, but should be avoided if possible.

Medical Referral

It has been seen that, although not many cases of superfluous hair are linked with physical illness, any excessive hair growth is in some way influenced by the endocrine system. Hormonal fluctuations, some natural and some artificial—if caused by such things as the Pill, fertility drugs, or hormonal therapy in the menopause—may cause hair growth to change in character.

If the operator suspects that the client's hair growth condition is due to an abnormal hormonal imbalance, then it may be necessary to refer her to her own doctor for a medical opinion. The speed of the change in the hair growth, the client's age, drug medication taken and her circumstances (for example, pre- or post-pregnancy), will all help the electrologist to decide whether she needs medical guidance to resolve the problem.

In many cases, this medical referral will simply act to confirm what is obvious: that the condition is hormonally linked, but falls within the band of hormonal alteration classed as 'normal'—that is, causing only side effects such as unwanted hair, which can be removed by electrology, and not requiring any specific medical treatment.

In some cases, vital medication, essential to the client's health, is known to produce unwanted hair as a side effect. This, however, is the price the individual has to pay for her overall health. Hormone therapy, such as is given during the menopause, is also known to have caused unwanted hair in predisposed women. Fertility drugs, prescribed for short periods to achieve conception in infertile women, can produce the same effects. Contraceptive drugs, the Pill, etc., can also increase hair growth on predisposed young women to an unacceptable level.

Medical referral may be sought broadly for two reasons: either to confirm what the client tells the operator about her physical condition, or to discover more about the client's condition and how it will affect the epilation treatment organization and progress. It has been seen that these internal forces can alter the hair growth, making it slow to respond to treatment and, in some cases, causing treatment difficulties, poor skin healing, and so on. If more hair is growing than the treatment can ever remove, the client is bound to be disappointed and may lose faith in her operator. It is, therefore, best for both the operator and the client to appreciate the problem fully, and to use medical help to reduce the hair growth potential if it is available.

Often the medical referral is purely a courtesy to the client's physician to advise him or her of what is planned and to ask for permission to treat the problem. (The client can undertake this task in most instances.) It does act as a safeguard by confirming that the treatment is not contra-indicated (unsuitable) for the client through a physical problem of which she is unaware.

CONTRA-INDICATIONS

There are a few conditions under which epilation is contra-indicated or where epilation would be contra-indicated for a particular individual without written medical permission. These are outlined below.

Heart Conditions

If the client has a heart condition, such as *angina pectoris*, or has a *pacemaker heart regulator* fitted, it may be possible to provide epilation, but the form the treatment would take must be decided by the client's medical specialist, and might need to be undertaken under medical supervision in a hospital. Each client must be considered on an individual basis, and the electrologist must adapt her work to fit in with the medical recommendations for each client. Recent work on a patient in England by one of the country's leading electrologists, operating under the guidance and control of the patient's heart specialist, has shown that electrology is possible on an individual fitted with a pacemaker device. The patient was connected to an electrocardiogram which monitored every stage of the treatment, and application procedures were altered where necessary for the safety of the patient. However, this is really specialized work and not part of normal electrology.

Naturally, this only indicates that the treatment could be made possible for this one individual patient and does not necessarily suggest that other people fitted with pacemaker devices are suitable clients. So, in a *normal* clinical practice, clients with heart conditions or fitted with pacemakers are contra-indicated and medical referral is essential.

Epilepsy

Epilation is normally contra-indicated for clients suffering from epilepsy, either *grand mal* or *petit mal* because a frequency of current is used which could trigger off an epileptic attack, fits, unconsciousness, etc. If the client is taking controlling drugs for her condition, medical approval may be given for epilation, with recommendations concerning methods of giving the treatment, duration of sessions, intensity levels of current and so on. There is, however, always the chance of an attack occurring during treatment, and, therefore, even if medical permission is granted, it is up to the operator to decide whether she wishes to undertake the treatment. The decision would depend on the electrologist's experience, and whether she felt able to cope with an epileptic fit, if one did occur. The client's own attitude and need for the treatment would inevitably play a large part in the operator's decision to help her.

Diabetes

Epilation is contra-indicated for clients suffering from *diabetes mellitus*, unless medical permission is given, because diabetics have particular problems with their skin. It is unstable, slow to replace itself, and healing is usually poor. Eruptions may occur after epilation treatment, and skin infection is a real hazard, requiring the use of meticulous pre- and home-care measures. Use of ozone therapy to disinfect the skin and improve healing, by steaming before and after each treatment can be very beneficial here. The diabetic client's skin is more subject to trauma than a normal skin, and pigmentation could occur after treatment if normal current intensities were used. So, the treatment has to be adjusted—low intensities used, probes very well spaced, treatment sessions short to avoid skin reactions, and appointments well spaced to allow for healing to take place.

Acne Vulgaris

Epilation is also contra-indicated for the young acne sufferer, unless medical permission is given, and even then a lot of problems present themselves when applying the treatment. The hormonal imbalance, which *causes* the increased activity of the sebaceous or oil glands resulting in the blemishes can also cause the growth of unwanted hair. In some cases the hairs are actually a major part of the skin eruptions, causing, as they grow, infection of the follicles, pustular conditions or deep-seated boils (see Chapter 6). The first step in treating hairs growing from infected follicles where pus is present is to use normal skin healing measures (for instance, ozone therapy, steaming) until the skin is clear, and only then commence epilation application. Stringent hygiene measures must be established with all instruments carefully sterilized before and after the application; skin cleansing measures should be thorough, but gentle; and healing, disinfecting lotions used throughout to settle the skin.

The acne skin is extremely sensitive and is prone to scarring or dark marking after the cautery. This hyperpigmentation is caused by alteration of the action of melanin cells in the area of the application as a result of the heat reaction. The exact stage of the acne condition should be noted on the client's record card at the start of the treatment, as well as any scarring already present, so that this cannot be attributed later to the epilation applications.

Ozone steaming plays a large part in the permissible treatment of the acne client, as it heals and disinfects and thus helps to bring the client to the stage where epilation is possible. In young men, who have to shave daily, impacted hairs are a real problem, for the skin can become raw and sore, as the pustules are opened each day by the razor. In some cases, the only way to cure these distorted hairs, which grow and curl back within the follicle, is to epilate them, curing the problem for good. Firstly, however, the infection has to be settled, in order to prevent it spreading and worsening the overall skin condition.

Treatment of acne sufferers, like diabetics, is more a question of treatment organization and good client co-operation, under medical direction, rather than special skill. It requires the most sympathetic handling, and although true overall success can be difficult to achieve the results are usually very worthwhile if the operator decides to take on the task.

Asthma

It is wise to be cautious when treating a client who tells you she suffers from asthma, as this is often a condition of nervous origin, suggesting that the client is highly strung, and suffers from nervous tension. Medical permission should be obtained prior to treatment, and the applications progressed cautiously until the client's capacity for treatment is known. Once the client feels secure in her treatment routine, and is not overstressed or anxious about it, it is likely that progress can be as normal. However, the operator should always be aware that she is dealing with an asthmatic who could have an attack, and should discuss with the client beforehand what steps should be taken if this should occur. Most asthmatics know exactly what they must do to help themselves, and it is usually simply a question of the electrologist understanding what is happening, and helping if necessary. It is to be recommended that an electrologist should have undergone First Aid training in order to provide her with knowledge and competence in the unlikely event of an accident or physical illness occurring.

If the difficult work is undertaken in liaison with medical practitioners, the operator can feel secure in the knowledge that she is looking after the best interests of her clients. She can seek guidance if she feels unsure about treating a client, she can receive confirmation of her opinion if she feels the client has a normally acceptable hormone imbalance, and she can avoid treating an unsuitable client for whom the treatment could be harmful.

It can also happen, although very rarely, that the electrologist is the first person to suspect a condition which requires medical attention. Changes in the form or growing rate of hair growth can be a valuable indicator of physical illness, and so electrologists have a responsibility to be especially vigilant. If the operator suspects that something might be amiss, she must tactfully, without causing anxiety, suggest that the client should consult her own doctor. It is not up to the electrologist to diagnose conditions for which she is not qualified, or cause alarm by stating what she thinks could be wrong. This is entirely outside the scope of the electrologist, but she can act in a sensible manner as a monitor if the possibility of an abnormality is present.

Pain Threshold

It has been seen that a client's capacity for epilation can be enhanced by many factors, including confidence in her surroundings, trust in the electrologist's abilities and knowledge, and faith that she can provide the solution to the client's problem. To these feelings of confidence and trust may be added techniques which can further relieve discomfort and alleviate tension and anxiety and so reduce the pain level.

As we have noted earlier, the electrologist should be sympathetic in her handling of the client, and at the same time confident in her expectation of solving the problem and decisive in mapping out the proposed treatment organization. However, it is wise to be responsive to the needs of the client here. Fitting the appointments to the client's personal circumstances and pocket, aids in gaining the client's co-operation in the treatment programme, and helps develop a mutual understanding between the professional and her client. The electrologist should be adaptable to the client's needs if she hopes to gain and keep her on a long-term basis. In fact, with some treatment programmes spanning over several years in severe or stubborn cases, clients become like old friends, and a very pleasant treatment atmosphere develops—free from tension and pain for the client.

The nature of the work itself prohibits much conversation being either possible or desirable during treatment, but some kind of interchange is necessary in order to be aware of the client's needs and feelings and hence to know how to adapt the application—when to work and when to pause, how to space the probes, and what adjustments to make to the current—to minimize the client's pain and maximize the results. This sympathetic awareness does a great deal to increase the client's capacity for treatment, and it relies not only on verbal exchange, but also on observation of the client's skin, her physical tension and response to the epilation application. In many cases, nothing is said between the operator and her client, rather it is *sensed* if the operator is in tune with her client's feelings.

Use of the fingers in skin contact not only aids the probe and application, but also provides feedback to the operator in terms of the client's tension, how she is coping with the discomfort and how close to her own pain-bearing level or pain threshold she is. Experienced operators can always tell when the client has had enough, and when to continue could cause distress. Sometimes the operator will be aware of this before the client, who may want to carry on doggedly with the treatment in order to make as much progress as possible.

Some clients who are very anxious to be rid of their hair problems can, on occasions, work against the end result by attempting to pressure the operator into applying treatment sessions too close together and thus preventing sufficient time for the healing of the subcutaneous skin layers to take place. This, as we have seen, can result in dehydration, pitting and scarring of the skin, and is therefore not in the client's best interests. If the underlying skin is not healed, the client will also feel more discomfort during subsequent applications in this area, the skin will react more visibly with instant reddening and swelling and there will be more danger of surface burns. In the end, this 'pushing in' of treatment is pointless, because long pauses will have to be added to the programme to allow the skin to recover fully, and overall progress will be slowed down.

Directing the client's attention *away* from the discomfort is possible, and some clinics have done this successfully by placing a varied assortment of interesting items close to the client's line of vision. This means, of course, that clients do not use eye pads—which many of them find claustrophobic anyway—but can look around and concentrate their attention on an interesting item, perhaps on a wall, rather than on the sensation being experienced.

Clients also find that being competently and firmly handled makes them feel secure and 'in good hands'. The operator's touch, when placing the client on the couch, or repositioning her to improve the probing application, should be gentle, but sure. The client should have the impression that the operator is guiding her throughout the entire application, initially by positioning her for treatment, then repositioning her during the application and finally helping her at the conclusion of the session.

Thus, this caring and positive attitude on the part of the electrologist helps increase the client's capacity for treatment and raises her pain threshold by reducing anxiety and tension, and also ensures her full co-operation in planning and carrying out the treatment programme.

TREATMENT ORGANIZATION

Epilation is a treatment of short application sessions which requires excellent treatment organization in order to be efficient. Operators must ensure that valuable time is not wasted during the appointment, otherwise the client will not receive a fair return for the money spent. If the operator is booked with continuous appointments, she must tidy up as she works, so as to be ready for each client as she arrives. Clients should be encouraged to arrive a little while before their appointment, not only to save time but also to enable them to settle down and become calm. It is not only very difficult to work well on a client who has rushed for an appointment and is tense and strung up, but her capacity for epilation will be poor. It is preferable to proceed with the next client, if she is present, and try to readjust appointments to fit in the late-comer when she arrives.

Clients are normally very reliable about keeping epilation appointments, as they are keen to resolve their hair problems and recognize the importance of regular attendance to the success of the treatment. Clients can either be given cards to remind them of their appointments, or they can attend at a regular time each week, fortnight, or month, depending on the treatment being undertaken. A regular appointment is usually easier for clients to remember and once they become accustomed to it they seldom miss it. This system helps the electrologist as well, as she is able to build up a regular clientele around these fixed appointments, and they form the backbone of her business. As most clients attend only once a fortnight or even once every three weeks, many clients are needed to provide the operator with a full practice.

Timing of Appointments and Treatment Adaptation

It has been seen that the hair condition—its strength, density, location, etc.—and the skin's sensitivity together determine the course the treatment will take. The skin acts as the limiting factor at all times, and it is around its capacity to heal and recover from epilation that appointments are planned. If extensive epilation is to be concentrated on **one small area** such as the upper lip, two weeks should be allowed between appointments. If healing proves to be good, this can be reduced to ten days in some cases; while in difficult or hypersensitive skin, three weeks may be needed to permit complete healing.

If the growth to be treated is ranged over **several areas**, these can be worked in rotation. Careful clinic records *must* be kept to ensure that an area is not treated a second time before its healing time has elapsed. As the skin often *appears* to be completely back to normal long before the *underlying* skin tissue has recovered, a written record must be kept to prevent further treatment being given prematurely.

If a **large area** of hair growth has to be treated, longer appointments can be given in order to make more progress. The only limitations here are the client's pain capacity, finances and available time. Hair growth covering the lip, chin and throat areas can be worked systematically to clear the whole area gradually, first thinning out the hairs and eventually rendering the follicles incapable of further growth. This is the most effective way in which to treat heavy growth, as the probes can be well spaced, and skin recovery is good, despite intensive epilation application. However, if clients prefer to concentrate on one area at a time and to remove the remaining hairs by temporary methods, then epilation is concentrated on a small area, and treatment sessions must again be given at two week intervals. This understandable wish to retain a groomed appearance while epilation is in progress can be a real problem to treatment organization. Nevertheless, it can be resolved by careful planning and co-operation between the client and the operator. Areas of facial growth can be left to grow in rotation, and disguised by a thin covering of tinted foundation make-up to avoid embarrassment. The hairs do not need to be very long for epilation, simply long enough to show follicle direction and allow the operator to remove them with the forceps. If the hairs are too short, probing will be slow and removals poor, so the client must understand the need for this small amount of growth. Because of this, however, at times certain adjustments may have to be made in the schedule to allow a normal social life to continue.

If clients are very embarrassed by their hair condition, and really cannot face life with visible hairs during the epilation programme, treatment can be organized in such a way as to prevent distress. These clients can be treated on a Monday having had the weekend for the hair to grow sufficiently to make treatment possible. They can then cut the remaining hairs after treatment, in order to be clean and able to face the world till the next appointment. Often hair growth is so strong than even two or three days gives the electrologist sufficient growth to work on. This is a slow and difficult way to perform epilation, but for a small proportion of clients it is the only way, and unless electrologists are adaptable they will lose these clients. For some individuals to have to admit to a hair problem is embarrassing in the extreme, so to expect them to allow the hairs to grow and show may be expecting the impossible.

A good time for a course of **leg hair epilation** or **inside thigh work** is the winter, when legs are usually covered up, and any skin spotting can be disguised by tights or trousers. Clients with a severe hair growth problem will probably be unused to showing off their legs, and so the effects of treatment will not disturb them unduly. However, for fashion-conscious young women having epilation for convenience, this is a point that should be borne in mind. The normal reaction to either the inside thigh or leg hair work is tiny brown spots, red or blue blood spots and occasionally scabbing if the growth has been extremely strong. In addition, work can proceed more easily and far faster if the hairs are left untouched. Thus, the hair situation is untidy, the skin is often temporarily marked, and, until the treatment programme is complete, the client is not likely to feel very well groomed. Since it can take as much as a year or two to remove leg hairs completely, it may be necessary to provide gaps in the treatment programme for holidays and other occasions when an immaculate appearance is desirable.

This need for treatment adaptation is another reason why it may not always be possible to know exactly how much a treatment will cost the client.

Treatment for leg and body hairs can be organized into half hour, one hour or even two hour appointments if the client is able to tolerate such long periods of treatment. One hour appointments at least are needed in order to make any impression on a large area such as the legs. If long appointments are booked, it is advisable to allow a short break in the middle of the appointment for a little rest, conversation and perhaps a cup of tea or coffee. This break not only helps to alleviate the strain on the client, but also to enhance the electrologist's concentration and thus the quality of her work.

Treatment on **very sensitive areas**, such as the breasts or abdomen, or on difficult areas such as the eyebrows or throat, are organized on a time basis, with the operator deciding how much can be accomplished during the period. Often half an hour is necessary, because of the difficulty of probing, and the need for slow and careful work. Treatment of these areas is classed as 'advanced work', and as such may cost more per hour than leg hair epilation, and possibly as much as facial epilation or advanced minor cosmetic electrology.

Because the true extent of a hair growth problem and the time needed to resolve it can only be ascertained on actual *inspection* of the condition, clients who telephone for advice should be advised to attend for a consultation, or sent an explanatory leaflet which explains the process of epilation and some of the factors which determine the progress of the treatment. These leaflets can be a great time saver to the busy practitioner, preventing long explanations over the phone in the midst of a busy day's work. The client can simply be sent a leaflet and invited to attend at a certain time for a consultation. This saves a lot of repetition and presents a very professional approach.

CLINIC RECORDS

It has already been seen that accurately recorded details of the client's hair condition should be made at the start of the treatment programme (see Chapter 1).

Medical History

In addition, a brief medical history should be entered to record whether a client is suitable for treatment, or whether epilation is contra-indicated and medical referral is advisable to determine the cause of the problem. This personal history should be obtained tactfully by explaining the need for it to the client.

GYNAECOLOGICAL DETAILS

The client's gynaecological history should be outlined briefly: pregnancies, miscarriages, surgical operations such as removal of a cyst on the ovaries or a hysterectomy (total removal of the womb), and hormone therapy received in the past or still being taken as this is very relevant to changes in hair growth.

Hormone Therapy

One of the female hormones, oestrogen, given to help middle-aged women through the menopause or 'change of life', often appears to reduce the incidence of unwanted hair, so common at this stage of life. Yet hormone therapy, given as a replacement for normal hormonal output following total removal of the womb and ovaries in the younger woman, has the opposite effect, causing unwanted hair to grow. However, its other benefits to the young woman deprived of her normal hormonal secretions are many, and enable her to live a full and healthy life. So some unwanted hair growth in pre-disposed females seems a relatively small price to pay for health.

Clients taking oral contraceptives—the Pill—to avoid pregnancy may find that they develop an increased density of hair in certain areas, such as the upper lip and chin. Therefore, a record of this hormone control should be made, together with the length of time the client has been on the Pill. It may perhaps be possible for the client to change the type of oral contraceptive she takes after discussion with her doctor. If the client receives contraceptive advice from a family planning clinic, then she may need to seek further advice from a doctor on the problem of her increased hair growth. Although many young women do seem rather pre-disposed to hair problems when on the Pill, it is a fact seldom discussed beforehand. It *is* a very common problem, and electrologists should be aware of it and advise their clients to seek medical help where necessary.

OTHER CONTRA-INDICATED CONDITIONS

Other physical conditions where epilation is contra-indicated and medical permission should be sought before treatment is undertaken are:

diabetes;
thyroid abnormalities;
heart conditions;
blood pressure problems;
epilepsy;
asthma.

In any event, medical guidance is needed, even if permission has been given, to devise the best method of treatment to ensure good results.

Treatment Record

The clinic card also provides a treatment record, listing the details of all epilation applications: the area treated, the length of the applications, the intensity level and the epilation unit used. This helps to prevent overtreatment of an area or premature re-treatment in any one area of the face or body.

In addition, the clinic record serves as a monitor of the client's *overall* progress, providing a complete record of the actual hours of work completed by the operator and paid for by the client. If a course of treatment does not appear to be providing the desired results and improvement, then the electrologist and client can check back on the number of sessions attended and make a comparison between the results expected and the results achieved in the given time. It may be that irregular attendance on the part of the client is to blame, or that the client has the wrong impression of the number of hours actually received and paid for. It is also possible that examination of the clinic records will point to a need to reassess the treatment programme or even to seek medical guidance in overcoming the hair growth problem.

Any client receiving hormone therapy treatment must be closely monitored and, if results are poor, with more hair growing than is being removed for instance, medical assistance must be sought. The electrologist can either write to the client's doctor or phone during a quiet period to ask for professional guidance, stating the problem encountered in resolving the superfluous hair condition. It may be possible for the hormone medication dosage to be altered to reduce the hair problem, while still achieving the necessary effect. If this is not possible, at least the client can be made aware of the reason for the slow progress, and her faith in the treatment will be retained.

Discussion between the client and operator on progress, or lack of it, shows a mutual understanding and a common goal, and builds up a feeling of trust which is essential in remedial epilation. Few electrologists would be in the business if they did not care about their clients, and medical referral as a part .of treatment organization illustrates this caring very clearly to the client.

CLINIC HYGIENE

The main concern when considering clinic hygiene is how to promote and maintain a state of cleanliness sufficient to prohibit the growth of bacteria. This state is known as *asepsis*.

Wet Sterilization

Asepsis can be obtained by washing down all available surfaces—walls, floors, couch, work surfaces, basins—after basic cleaning with an antiseptic solution such as Dettol or Savlon concentrates, diluted down according to the manufacturer's instructions to a level to suit the task in hand. Towels can also be sterilized by this method, as can epilation tools. If metal tools are sterilized using this cold water method, care must be taken to use a glass container and a rust inhibiting factor. Instrument Dettol, Cetavlon (zephiran chloride) or a similar solution can be used, made up to the correct dilution and *changed every day*. This is important in order to be assured of effective sterilization.

Vapour Sterilization

Metal and plastic tools can also be sterilized using vapour sterilization methods. This is done in wall or trolley cabinets, which also provide sterile storage for the items, using formaldehyde and heat to achieve sterilization. However, the metal tools must be clean and dry before being placed in the cabinet, otherwise they will rust. It is also worthwhile covering the shelves with cotton gauze to absorb moisture from the tools and prevent damage.

Ultraviolet sterilization

Ultraviolet sterilization can also be used, again in closed wall or trolley cabinets, but this time electrically powered.

If the tools are clean, free from skin debris and dry, complete sterilization can be achieved in only twenty minutes, no matter which method—wet, vapour or ultraviolet—is used.

Autoclave sterilization

Another, less common, but very effective method is heat sterilization using an autoclave sterilizer. (This method is commonly used by dentists.) In recent times, problems of cross-infection of diseases transmitted through the use of needles in acupuncture has highlighted the need for more reliable sterilization procedures. This is particularly important in electrology where work does not usually take place under medical supervision, and a client suffering from an infectious disease might quite possibly be treated. Cross-infection—the passing of infection from one client to another through the needles—might then occur if there had been inadequate sterilization. Several serious diseases can be transmitted in this way, including hepatitis (jaundice), and therefore effective needle sterilization is very important. Where the disposable sterilized needles *Sterex* are available, these are the obvious first choice, providing a new sterile needle for each client, leaving small tools only to be autoclaved. Up to now electrology has had a very good record for hygiene, but the profession must always be alert to possible improvements. The autoclave sterilizer is one of these, and it is possible that the medical and public health authorities will make it a compulsory piece of equipment in the future.

The autoclave sterilizer works on the vapour sterilization principle. The unit consists of two chambers: water is placed in the lower chamber and the tools in the chamber above it. The unit is then closed. The water is boiled and steam released into the upper chamber for about ten to twenty minutes. The sterilized items are then removed with forceps and placed in a closed glass container until required. In a busy clinic, several sets of forceps and a selection of needles are needed for a day's work, and these can all be sterilized together, with the small items being loosely wrapped in gauze to prevent loss. (Plastic items cannot be sterilized by this method as the heat level would cause them to melt; they must be treated by the cold water, vapour or ultraviolet methods.)

It is the needles which pose the greatest problem for the electrologist, and use of disposable sterile needles seems the ideal solution, with the use of the autoclave sterilizer for all small metal tools (and needles, if *Sterex* are not available). It is up to electrologists to seek out their solutions to sterility—it is their livelihood at stake.

Short Wave Diathermy Current Sterilization

Another, very common method of sterilizing needles is to heat them just prior to the epilation application by using the short wave diathermy current from the epilation unit at a high intensity. This has appeared to be a satisfactory solution up to now. However, many epilation units these days do not provide sufficient power for completely effective sterilization. Although electrologists will continue to use the diathermy current to clean (by running the tweezers along the length of the needle) and sterilize the needle *during* applications, a more realible method of sterilization *between* applications now seems necessary. This may not be because professional electrologists themselves are less vigilant, but because of the less clinical, and therefore less hygienic, circumstances in which electrology is offered these days—in department stores and beauty salons, for instance.

Individual or Disposable Needles

The modern way to avoid the need for elaborate needle sterilization (which always contains the element of human error) is to change to disposable sterile needles, *Sterex*. The client has a brand new needle each treatment, which is charged to her directly, or costed into the treatment charge. Once used, those needles are thrown away after treatment—ideally into a special *Sharp's* container, to avoid the risk of cross-infection.

The disposable *Sterex* needles are presently of the Ferrie type, in a range of diameters, individually packed, and available in boxes of 50 of each size. They are gamma-irradiated—just like hypodermics—in batches, whereupon yellow dots on the individual needle packets turn red. This indicates they are sterile. They are put into the needle holder in a special way to avoid finger contact, using the little plastic tube which protects the needle tip, to position them correctly into the needle holder. So the client gets a perfect sterile needle every time—a real advance in treatment.

General Hygiene

Apart from the methods of promoting a sterile environment outlined above, a number of other precautionary measures should be used to reduce the risk of infection:

(1) Disposable tissues and paper sheets should be used.

(2) Clean towels must be provided for each client. These should be boiled if they have been used in connection with a skin infection such as acne.

(3) Instruments should be sterilized after cleaning and kept in a closed, sterile cabinet when not in use.

(4) The operator must wash her hands before and after each treatment.

Maintenance of Hygiene

If the clinic, working position, tools and other equipment are clean and sterile to begin with, maintaining asepsis simply means being vigilant about standards of hygiene during the day's work. It is pointless to start off in a hygienic fashion if this is not maintained by attention to cleanliness during epilation practice.

Towels, tissues and paper sheeting and other equipment must be stored in a clean manner and disposed of immediately after use—either thrown away or placed for washing outside the working area. Cotton-wool, tissues and other items used in cleaning and epilation procedures must be placed in a covered waste receptacle, which should be emptied between clients. No soiled cotton-wool or gauze pieces should be left on the trolley between treatments, but should be disposed of as they are used. Cotton-wool pieces, gauze, lotions, creams and other materials should all be kept in closed conainers, clean and ready for use. Anything accidently dropped on the floor should either be thrown away, or resterilized.

If the operator has a cold and needs to pause to blow her nose, she should move away from the client and, after blowing her nose, should wash her hands before resuming treatment. In this instance, a face mask made of gauze and covering the operator's nose and mouth, can be worn to prevent the spreading of germs to the client. The magnifier does act as a breath shield but the close proximity of operator and client during treatment inevitably means that there is a high risk of passing on an infection.

CLIENT CARE

Client care has already been considered in terms of being responsive to the client's feelings, reassuring about the outcome of treatment and improving treatment capacity by skilful and caring handling and conversation. These psychological aspects of care, however, need to be reinforced by physical measures to minimize skin damage while achieving satisfactory results. After assessing the skin's capacity for epilation during the consultation and initial treatment, a programme of pre- and aftercare treatment should be worked out, to be backed up by home-care measures. If the skin is hypersensitive, slow to heal, or shows some other problem, special precautions will be needed to avoid skin infection or other damage. Even with normal skins, careful precare and aftercare steps will help advance the progress of the treatment programme and prevent skin marking, scarring or pigmentation problems from arising.

Precare

Epilation should be performed on a really clean skin, of normal temperature, prepared with a soothing lotion to cool the skin's surface and reduce the risk of inflammation or swelling following epilation. If make-up is worn, it must be removed gently, in order to avoid stimulating the surface capillaries, which would result in increased skin reaction to epilation. Antiseptic solutions should not be used on the skin as these can be very irritating to the surface tissues. Rather, lotions which soothe the skin, both by their coolness and anti-inflammatory ingredients, should be used. Each electrologist will have her own favourite solutions for use on the skin during treatment. Many of them are based on flower, plant or herbal extracts known for their soothing effects: camomile lotions, solutions based on tincture of benzoin (light tincture of benzoin), and elder-flower lotions, all have elements which soothe and settle the skin, so aiding healing. Many of these ingredients are also anti-inflammatory and reduce swelling, thus helping to avoid some of the worst effects of epilation treatment. When these lotions are used both before and during treatment, the skin stays calm, and more treatment can be performed without skin distress. Some operators prefer to use a very diluted skin antiseptic such as Savlon, because they feel that it reduces the risk of any skin infection. However, the skin is very capable of healing itself, given the right conditions, such as cleanliness during treatment and protection after treatment to avoid bacterial invasion of the follicle.

As long as a preparation lotion does not coat or block the skin, making probing difficult, and is not a skin irritant or caustic in nature, it can be used for soothing the skin.

One recipe which has proved very successful with many electrologists is based on light tincture of benzoin (to promote healing), elder-flower water (for anti-inflammatory effect) and tincture of myrrh (a gum resin which appears to help in the healing process and acts like a preservative). All these ingredients can be obtained in small quantities through a pharmacist or chemist, and can easily be made up into the soothing solution in the clinic using ordinary household utensils.

Recipe for Soothing Lotion

Ingredients:
2 dessert spoons elder-flower water
½oz (14g) simple or light tincture of benzoin

10 drops tincture of myrrh
just under 1pt (less than 0.5 litre) water

Method:

Place the elder-flower in a bottle and first add the water and then the tincture of benzoin. The lotion will become cloudy. Then add ten drops of tincture of myrrh, place the top on the bottle, and give the mixture a good shake. Small bottles for trolley use can then be filled; these should preferably be made of glass, as the tincture of benzoin produces a brown deposit which can discolour plastic bottles, making them look dirty and unpleasant. The bulk lotion should be shaken each time before the trolley bottles are refilled, as the suspension settles to the bottom and the effective ingredients are, therefore, not evenly spread through the solution. The smell will indicate whether the solution is the correct strength. If it is, the lotion will have a pleasant, rather clinical smell, and will feel instantly cooling and soothing to the skin. If not, it should be diluted down with water until the correct strength is achieved. The lotion does not need refrigeration, but must be kept in a cool place to prolong its effectiveness. Keeping the bulk lotion in a brown glass bottle helps to prolong the active nature of the ingredients, but again this is not essential.

Many electrologists use this lotion in their work, and find it answers most purposes. It can be used to prepare clean skin, soothe skin during treatment and to conclude the routine. In most cases of body epilation, it is all that is required, although on the face more camouflaging and protective measures may be required after treatment.

Aftercare

The preparation needed for aftercare of the skin following epilation must be protective, antibacterial in nature to prevent infection and can be flesh tinted for skin camouflage. Calamine based creams are often used. Calamine itself is a soothing ingredient which is well known for its cooling effect on erythema (reddening of the skin and increased skin temperature). It achieves this effect by vasoconstriction of the capillaries close to the skin's surface, and so is an ideal aftercare preparation following the trauma of epilation. Many preparations also have an antihistamine ingredient which reduces skin swelling and inflammation. Creams and lotions are available under a variety of brand names; *Caladryl* is a well-known preparation in Europe.

Any medicated powder can also provide protection and, through its drying effect, speed the healing process. Flesh-coloured tinted powders, such as *Eckosan* powder, are very effective, providing both protection and camouflage in the one application. If one medicated powder is difficult to obtain, a pharmacist will often be able to recommend a substitute. Multi-purpose powders, such as foot powders or preparations for nappy rash, designed not only to dry and heal, but also to prevent the increase of bacteria, can often be used. These powders can be used both as an aftercare measure and also at home between epilation appointments if necessary. Clients with skin healing problems, hypersensitive skin, or a severe hair growth condition may have to be advised to use protective products on their skin to avoid infection, applying them as a normal part of skin care at home. They can be used under normal make-up, after the first day or two following treatment, to act as a buffer between the skin and the make-up, and to further the skin healing process.

Many electrologists simply use their soothing lotion as an aftercare measure, and rely on the skin to heal itself if kept clean and allowed to settle naturally. If lotion alone is used after treatment, the client must be advised not to wash the area until the following day, allowing twenty-four hours for the skin to recover without interference. If the epilation technique has been good enough and the skin shows very little adverse effect following treatment, then by the next day no sign of a reaction to the application should remain, and the skin can be treated as normal. Each epilated hair follicle will by that time have started to heal naturally at its base, and no external sign of the treatment should be evident. The skin does rely, however, on a meticulous approach to initial protection and cleanliness following treatment. Therefore, co-operation from the client on home-care is extremely important.

Home-care

In nearly every case where skin healing is poor, the reason will be found to be interference with the skin by the client following the application. This may be due either to poor explanation of the home-care measures required, or simply to lack of co-operation on the part of the client. It has been seen previously how vital is the client's co-operation in ensuring treatment success, and home-care is no exception in this respect.

If the client is aggravating the skin between

epilation treatments, or simply not following a hygienic routine, skin healing will be poor and the risk of skin dehydration, pitting, marking and pigmentation problems will be increased. If clients understand that skin protection is needed to avoid skin infection, their co-operation is far more likely to be forthcoming.

The client must be advised to leave the skin alone for as long as possible after treatment in order to allow it to settle and return to normal skin temperature. Lotions or creams will have been applied to the skin following epilation, and these should be left in place, ideally, until the day following the treatment. By this time, the skin's normal healing processes will have taken over the task of skin recovery.

If the client is very conscious of her appearance and feels the need for camouflage, she should be provided with tinted calamine creams or flesh-tinted powders of a medicated type. It should be emphasized that *make-up should on no account be applied immediately following epilation*: skin infection can easily result. Clients who normally wear tinted foundations, however, may revert to these twenty-four hours after treatment, but should still apply the protective product prior to applying the make-up. The electrologist should also make it absolutely clear that make-up preparations should be removed very carefully in order to avoid aggravating the skin and inducing infection. It is advisable to discuss with the client any products likely to be used for skin care and make-up between treatments to be sure that nothing will be used which might delay skin healing. Hypo-allergenic preparations are very gentle in action, and are to be recommended for use on skin undergoing a programme of epilation treatment.

Temporary Removal Methods during Epilation Programme

It is quite likely that clients will wish to remove offending hairs by some temporary method during the epilation programme. It is therefore essential to gain the client's co-operation in using the correct method of temporary hair removal—that is, *cutting* the hairs—and this can best be achieved by offering an explanation of the effects that depilatory products have on the skin and the consequence of plucking and waxing unwanted hairs.

EFFECTS OF CHEMICAL DEPILATORIES

The surface of the skin is continually being shed (desquamated) from its horny layers, and chemical depilatories accelerate this process while removing the unwanted hairs. Depilatories act by dissolving the hairs, and since both the stratum corneum and the hair shaft are composed of the same hard keratin, they are both dissolved by the depilatory product. This leaves the skin's most superficial layer considerably thinner and more exposed, and more susceptible to bacterial invasion. The protective function of the skin is thus considerably reduced, and irritation, allergic reactions and dermatitis are more likely to occur. The skin's capacity to cope with trauma or injury is reduced, and healing becomes slow and difficult. The skin may also suffer from pigmentation abnormalities while healing is taking place, and brown marks may appear as a result of a heat reaction on the sensitive tissue.

EFFECTS OF PLUCKING OR WAXING

Plucking or waxing of unwanted hairs can cause distortion of the follicles, which in turn can result in abnormal hair growth.

Continual plucking does appear to increase the *strength of the growth* in some individuals, resulting in the formation of deeper follicles which are very difficult to probe accurately. This increased strength may be brought about by increased vascular activity of the tiny blood vessels which encapsulate the follicle down its length, caused by the follicle's constant need to replace the forcibly removed hair.

Experience does seem to show that hairs that are continually plucked or waxed also increase their *rate of growth*. This may be an illusion however, brought about by the fact that all hairs have been brought to the same stage in the growth pattern, and all regrow at once (whereas only a percentage of hairs would normally be in the anagen or active stage, while others would be resting or in the process of transition or change).

In any event, the plucking of strong hairs is pointless, offering no permanent solution to the hair problem, and should be discontinued while epilation treatment is in progress. Waxing has a similar effect to plucking, but is worse in that it affects *all* the hairs, fine vellus hairs as well as superfluous hairs.

The temptation to pluck out offending hairs is a real problem for clients, and operators must be aware of this and ready to suggest alternative means of removal if they hope to gain clients' co-operation.

In addition, every endeavour should be made

within the epilation programme to remove those hairs which are very apparent and a worry to the client. Naturally, this may only be possible if the skin is able to stand the treatment, and the probes do not need to be placed so close together that they will cause skin damage. It has been seen that probes must be well spaced in the early days of an electrologist's experience. But, even an experienced operator should place the probes one-tenth to one-eighth of an inch apart (2 to 3 mm), in order to permit healing and prevent overlap of heat reactions.

Electrologists must use their common sense as far as this aspect of treatment organization is concerned, and attempt to clear quickly as many offending hairs as possible, so leaving as few as possible as a temptation to the client. Then those hairs that have to remain till the next appointment can be closely cut off next to the skin. When treating elderly clients, it may be a kindness and a courtesy to perform this small task for them, if their eyesight is poor. They will feel much happier if they know they present a tidy appearance to the world.

In this way the operator can keep her clients content, gain their co-operation and at the same time get on with the job of epilation unrestricted or unhampered by skin problems.

OZONE AND VAPOUR STEAMING

Ozone steaming is found to be a beneficial aid to skin healing with young problem skins, dry sensitive skins and skin conditions, such as are found in diabetes, where healing is known to be poor. It can also be used where long sessions of extensive treatment are being given, or on any individual whose skin seems prone to infection or strong reaction.

Time has to be allowed for the application of ozone steaming before and after the epilation application, and this must naturally be costed into treatment charges. It can, however, make the difference between success and failure for a small percentage of clients, and therefore should be applied wherever it is indicated. Indeed, it can actually enable a client with a hypersensitive or problem skin to handle epilation successfully rather than have it contra-indicated, and so it does extend treatment possibilities in the clinic.

Ozone steaming is a natural means of activating the circulation of the subcutaneous vessels and providing them with oxygen. The *Vapozone* ap-

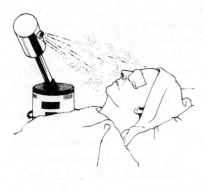

plication has a disinfecting, antibacterial action on skin tissue, which normalizes the acid/alkaline (pH) balance and promotes healing. Ozone is produced in the head of the equipment by means of a quartz tube, high-pressure mercury lamp, over which the water vapour passes and becomes ionized. The physiological actions include:

(1) the heating action of the ionized water vapour;
(2) the action of the ozone and its derivatives;
(3) the action of the ultraviolet radiation arising from decomposition of the ozone.

Slight perspiration is induced, the stratum corneum becomes hydrated and softened and desquamation (skin shedding) is increased. Ozone and the active oxygen produced by its decomposition destroy organic substances and bacteria. Furthermore, the increased blood circulation resulting from this action permits the effects of the ozone to act not only on the surface of the epidermis, but also in the cutaneous tissues.

Method of Application

The equipment should first be checked to ensure that there is a sufficient supply of purified water in the reservoir tank. Then, five to ten minutes before treatment is due to begin, it should be switched on to heat up the water; the vapour switch *only* is required at this stage. When it starts to discharge water vapour from the head of the equipment, the ozone control should be switched on to begin the production of ozone. The steam then becomes ionized and changes its consistency, assuming a very fine cloud-like appearance. At this time, crackling is heard from the vicinity of the quartz tube in the equipment head.

While the steamer is heating the water, the electrologist may prepare the client for the epilation treatment and cleanse the skin if necessary. It is advisable, at this stage, to explain the ozone treatment and its effects to the client, and prepare her for the unusual smell and noise of the apparatus. The eyes must be covered with damp cotton-wool pads to avoid irritation, and any areas of extreme sensitivity, such as the upper cheeks, protected with dry cotton-wool.

The client should be placed in a semi-upright position, and the fully operating steamer arranged so that it generates an *even* distribution of ionized vapour over the treatment area. The length of application time depends on the condition of the skin, and the following durations are only approximate:

(1) **Hypersensitive skins**—five minutes before

and after the epilation application at a distance of fifteen inches (38 cm) from the lip and chin area.

(2) **Dry sensitive skins**—five minutes before and five to ten minutes after the application (to promote healing) at a distance of ten to twelve inches (25 to 30 cm) from the facial area.

(3) **Acne skin conditions**—(for a disinfecting and antibacterial effect) ten minutes before and after the epilation application at a distance of ten inches (25 cm). In severe cases, the length of application time can be increased as necessary, and to avoid over-reaction the distance from the skin can be increased. Operators must keep a close watch on the reaction of the skin, both during the application, and after the epilation treatment, and then use their own judgement to determine how much ozone steaming will prove beneficial.

(4) **Diabetic conditions**—there are no firm guidelines for the use of ozone therapy on diabetic skins. It should be used as needed, varying the time and distance according to the state of the skin. The diabetic skin is very unstable and suffers from periodic out-breaks of skin eruptions, which ozone steaming can help to settle. The skin may stand up to epilation treatment very well, and then suddenly appear to suffer from a severe reaction, with skin irritation, blemishes, and areas of unhealed, sore skin. The skin can then be helped back to normality by ozone steaming and careful home-care measures.

The amount of ozone steaming that can be applied, like the amount of epilation, depends entirely on the state of the skin at the time. However, the following can be used as a general guideline. As a precautionary measure to help the skin cope with the trauma of epilation, five minutes ozone steaming can be applied before and after epilation, at a distance of twelve to fifteen inches (30 to 38 cm). If the skin is in a rather sensitive condition, with high colour and obvious irritation, ozone steaming can be applied ten minutes before and after epilation at fifteen inches (38 cm) distance. If the skin is in a really distressed condition, and epilation is temporarily contra-indicated, ozone steaming can be applied independently for twenty minutes at a distance of twelve to fifteen inches (30 to 38 cm) to help skin recovery.

Chapter 5

Causes of Superfluous Hair Growth. The Endocrine System

Unwanted hair can be divided into two categories: 'normal' and 'abnormal' growth. Normal hair growth is that due to genetic or racial factors which predispose the individual to a heavy hair growth. Abnormal hair growth is that which is directly associated with endocrine influence which causes changes in the hormonal balance of the body and so alters the hair growth. It is important that the electrologist knows whether the hair growth presented to her for treatment is normal or abnormal, as this will determine the treatment that should be adopted and the progress that can be expected. It may also indicate whether medical advice should be sought. Although very little of the electrologist's work will be considered to be on abnormal growth, that is connected with physical illness, in a sense all hair growth that deviates from the normal pattern is abnormal, and can be attributed to endocrine influence.

The hair can be thought of as an 'end organ' of the endocrine system, and as such responds to minute alterations in its internal secretions, carried by hormonal messages through the bloodstream. These internal stimuli can cause the hairs to change in character, grow weaker or stronger, disappear altogether, or grow in an excessive form.

Malfunction of or alterations in the endocrine system also bring about physical change, altering body weight, skin colour, texture and temperature, and these changes, in addition to the changes in hair growth, act as pointers to the cause of the condition. Electrologists may well find themselves working in conjunction with the medical world in treating abnormal hair growth and will, therefore, need to have a basic knowledge of the endocrine system and its effect on the body.

The *structure* of the follicle and hair has already been considered in detail, and it has been noticed that in this knowledge lies the key to reversal of the growth process—the hair destruction by epilation. Now, in order to attain a thorough understanding of hair *function*, it is necessary to consider briefly the endocrine system and its effects on hair growth, both in normal health and illness.

Before embarking on this, however, let us first consider the correct terminology for different types of superfluous hair and the underlying causes.

HYPERTRICHOSIS AND HIRSUTISM

Hypertrichosis and hirsutism (or hirsuties) are terms used to describe different hair growth conditions, and act as an indicator as to the likely cause of the problem.

Hypertrichosis is defined as a growth of coarse, terminal hair which is considered excessive for the age, sex and race of the individual. It is an overdevelopment of localized extent, and its causes are not always clear. However, the hair growth does *not* follow a male sexual pattern, and hypertrichosis is not considered to be androgen dependent.

Hirsutism is a condition of wider, general growth of excessive terminal hair in the *adult male sexual pattern*. It can be accompanied by other male-type characteristics, and is usually androgen induced, occurring in conditions where there is hormone imbalance, for example, tumour of the adrenal or pituitary glands, problems of ovarian origin, or the menopause.

As has been seen, all hair growth can to some extent be considered endocrine dependent, with the hair follicle thought of as an end organ of the endocrine system, responding to changes in the body caused by hormonal influence. Some of these changes occur as a result of normal stages in life, where hormonal activity is increased or in a process of change: adolescence, pregnancy and the menopause are all stages where the incidence of unwanted hair growth is increased. Excessive hair growth may also be an indicator of illness—for instance, the malfunction of certain glands (for example, the adrenal glands) or the presence of a cyst which is impairing the function and hormonal output of the ovaries.

The terms hypertrichosis and hirsutism are often interchanged, and, indeed, there are a lot of characteristics common to both conditions, although correctly only hair that grows in a male sexual pattern should be classed as hirsutism or hirsuties. The term *hirsute* has for so long been used as a description of general hairiness that no doubt it will continue to be used in this way. However, electrologists should be aware of the difference between the two conditions, in as much as one is an indicator of some abnormality that may need medical attention, while the other may simply be an inherent condition the client must learn to live with, and improve by professional help if possible.

Causes of Hypertrichosis

(1) Genetic or racial predisposition—hereditary tendency to heavy hair growth.
(2) Stress, anxiety and worry.
(3) Hormone imbalance:
    (a) Natural glandular changes (puberty, pregnancy and the menopause);
    (b) Disfunction or disease of certain endocrine glands (pituitary, thyroid or adrenal);
    (c) Tumour or cyst on certain glands;
    (d) Removal of certain glands (partial or complete hysterectomy, or the removal of one ovary);
    (e) Reaction to certain drugs (cortisone, testosterone).

Causes of Hirsutism

(1) Genetic, racial, family and individual predisposition.
(2) Problems of adrenal origin.
(3) Problems of ovarian origin.
(4) Sexual abnormalities.
(5) Systemic illness, i.e. Iatrogenic—Archard Thiers Syndrome.

Thus, it can be seen how similar are the causes of the two defined types of hair growth, and it is for this reason that medical guidance is so often required.

All hair growth, wherever it is found on the body, and whether normal or excessive, can be said to be hormone dependent. However, it is the beard area of facial hair, axillary, chest, abdominal and pubic hair that are classified as 'sexual hair', and *changes* involving these areas would point to hirsutism and the growth being androgen induced.

Hypertrichosis or hairiness does not normally follow this adult male sexual pattern, with its associated signs of virilism, but is more generalized in growth. A client may suffer from a severe hair problem, but be normal physically, suffering no ill effects from the growth other than mental distress. Many nationalities accept as normal a level of hair growth unacceptable to European taste, this hairiness being part of the racial characteristics, common to most females of that nationality. The hair growth may be *excessive*, but not *abnormal* for the racial type.

THE ENDOCRINE SYSTEM

A full study of the endocrine system is beyond the scope of this book, and unnecessary for the electrologist's purposes. Rather, it is important for her to have an understanding of the relationship between changes in the body caused by endocrine influence and their effect on hair growth patterns. For this purpose, a knowledge of the function of the endocrine system, and its effect on the body, is essential. The endocrine system does not operate independently, but interacts with other systems of the body to control bodily functions and maintain the physical equilibrium against changes in the environment.

From the science of neuroendocrinology, we know that the **hypothalamus** of the brain, which acts as master control of the endocrine system, is also the 'head Ganglion' of the autonomic nervous system.

Endocrine Glands

Endocrine glands are usually groups of cells without ducts which secrete directly into the bloodstream. They produce *hormones*, which are chemical messengers in the body and which help to control the metabolic functions of other cells and tissues. The chief endocrine glands are the **suprarenal** glands, the **thyroid** gland, the **parathyroid** glands, the **pituitary** gland (hypophysis cerebri) and **pineal** gland, while certain other organs have subsidiary endocrine functions, for example, the pancreas, the stomach, the small intestine, the ovaries, the testes and the placenta in pregnancy.

SUPRARENAL GLANDS OR ADRENAL BODIES

One of these glands lies capping each kidney. The glands are formed of *cortex* derived from the same tissue as the kidneys and the gonads, and *medulla* derived from the same tissue as the sympathetic cords.

Functions of the Suprarenal Glands

The **cortex** produces *adrenal cortical hormone* or *cortin*, which is essential to life. It contains a metabolic hormone, a salt and water hormone and sex hormones. The metabolic hormone is antagonistic to insulin like the glycotropic factor of the pituitary to which it is related. It affects the metabolism of fats, proteins and carbohydrates. The salt and water hormone controls the excretion of salt and water from the body. The sex hormones produced by the cortex are additional to those of the gonads, and probably account for the occurrence of small amounts of female hormones in men and male hormones in women.

The medulla produces *adrenaline* which stimulates the breakdown of glycogen in the liver and the muscles, thereby increasing the amount of sugar in the blood. It also increases blood pressure and the rate of the heartbeat, decreases the time taken for blood to clot and temporarily stops breathing. Production of adrenaline is increased by emotions such as fear and anger, and its action prepares the body for bursts of activity.

THYROID GLAND

The thyroid gland lies in the lower part of the neck, formed of two *lobes* connected by an isthmus, one lobe lying on each side of the trachea (windpipe). The lobes are composed of small closed *vesicles* lined by epithelium, containing gelatinous, colloidal material into which the gland's secretion, *thyroxin*, passes. The gland receives its blood supply from branches of the *carotid* and *subclavian arteries*, and is richly supplied with blood vessels, through which the hormone is eventually removed.

Functions of the Thyroid Gland

The gland produces a compound *thyroxin*, which contains iodine and helps control general metabolism. The thyroid gland interacts and co-operates with other ductless glands in the general endocrine balance of the body. It affects the irritability of the nervous system, and is intimately related to the condition of the skin and hair. Changes in the level of the thyroid gland's secretion—its under- or overactivity—quickly affect the nature of the hair growth and the texture of the skin. The thyroid gland stores iodine, and any malfunction of the gland which alters the level of secretion of thyroxin can cause physical and mental abnormalities in infants, limiting development and resulting in cretinism.

Oversecretion (or **hyperthyroidism**) results in increased metabolism, and affects the individual's weight, body temperature and speed of movements, making them appear thin, tense and nervous. This condition may be caused by a *goitre*, an enlargement of the gland which produces increased levels of hormonal secretion into the bloodstream, although it also has other endocrine-linked causes. Disorders of the thyroid gland linked with oversecretion are also known as *thyrotoxicosis*.

Undersecretion (or **hypothyroidism**) results in lower metabolic rate and increase in weight, and a tendency to slowness in speech, movements and mental processes. This condition, also known as *myxoedema*, brings about changes in the hair and skin, and superfluous hair is often a side effect of undersecretion of the thyroid. As previously mentioned, undersecretion in children can result in cretinism, where development is retarded and the child can appear mentally defective.

The thyroid hormones also increase the sensitivity of the body tissues to the effects of adrenaline secreted by the medulla of the suprarenal glands.

PARATHYROID GLANDS

The parathyroid glands are found lying close to the thyroid gland; they are four in number and small in size. The secretion of these glands is called *parathormone*; it controls the excretion of phosphates, and, therefore, indirectly controls the amount of calcium in the blood. It is the effects of the shortage or excess of calcium which are noticeable in parathyroid diseases.

PITUITARY GLAND OR HYPOPHYSIS CEREBRI

The pituitary gland lies in the *sella turcica* of the *sphenoid bone*, attached by a thin stalk to the hypothalamus at the base of the brain. The neural stalk and the neural lobe, or *pars nervosa*, develop from the brain of the embryo and constitute the *neurohypophysis*. The *pars anterior, pars intermedia* and *pars tuberalis* develop from the non-nervous tissue and constitute the *adenohypophysis*.

The terms *posterior lobe* and *anterior lobe* represent a morphological (or structural) division through the intra-glandular cleft which does not correspond with the division by origin or function.

Functions of the Pituitary Gland

The Neurohypophysis

This produces what is usually known as *posterior lobe* extract containing two distinct hormones: *oxytocin* and *vasopressin* (antidiuretic hormone—ADH).

Oxytocin causes contraction of the uterine and mammary smooth muscles, and so stimulates contraction of the uterus during birth and the release of milk during breast-feeding.

Vasopressin has a powerful effect on the reabsorption of water by the kidneys, and is therefore known as an antidiuretic hormone. It acts as a regulator, balancing the amount of fluid required by the body, and the rate of release of vasopressin is altered by changes in the blood's pressure, volume and flow. Other factors, such as pain, emotional stress, etc., also alter the rate of release of the hormone.

The Adenohypophysis

This is considered the master gland of the endocrine system, and produces anterior lobe extract with seven distinct effects attributed to separate hormones, most of them being classed as *trophic hormones.* The anterior lobe produces hormones which are instrumental in controlling the secretions of the other endocrine glands.

Somatotrophic hormone (STH) controls the growth of the body by controlling skeletal development. An excess of this hormone causes giantism in the young and acromegaly in adults, a condition where the bones, especially the long bones, become lengthened and distort the features, limbs and digits (fingers and toes). Deficiency of this hormone causes dwarfism.

Thyrotrophic hormone (TTH) governs the activity of the thyroid gland and production of thyroxin.

Adrenocorticotrophic hormone (ACTH) governs the secretion of some of the hormones produced by the adrenal cortex.

Follicle stimulating hormone (FSH) stimulates growth of ovarian follicles and the secretion of oestrogens in the female and spermatogenesis in the male. The gonadotrophic hormones are also involved in the formation and maintenance of the *corpora lutea* in women and the *seminiferous tissue in* men.

Luteinizing (or **interstitial cell stimulating hormone** (ICSH) controls the secretion of oestrogen and progesterone in the ovaries, and control secretion of testosterone in the testes.

Lactogenic hormone (LTH) (or **mammotrophin**) controls the secretion of milk during breast-feeding by stimulating the mammary glands. It also helps to maintain the *corpus luteum* during pregnancy.

Melanocyte stimulating hormone (MSH) causes an increase in cutaneous pigmentation.

Other factors attributed to the pituitary extract cannot be isolated as separate hormones, and include:

The ketogenic factor, which alters fat metabolism, thus changing the amount of ketone bodies in the blood and urine and transferring fat deposits from the body to the liver.

The glycotrophic factor, which acts as an antagonist to insulin.

The pancreatrophic factor, which increases the secretion of insulin by the islet cells in the pancreas, and, therefore, counteracts the action of the glycotrophic factor.

The diabetogenic factor, which in excess induces diabetes by destruction of the islet tissues.

The parathyrotrophic factor, which stimulates the parathyroid glands.

These five factors may result from an imbalance between the growth hormone and the adrenocorticotrophic hormone acting through the adrenal cortex.

PINEAL GLAND

The pineal gland or epiphysis cerebri is situated beneath the posterior part of the corpus callosum. It secretes melatonin into the bloodstream, being involved in the reproductive function.

Functions of the Hypothalamus

It has been seen that the hypothalamus is the master controller of the endocrine system and closely associated with the autonomic nervous system. It is now known that the controls exerted on the endocrine system and the lower autonomic centres by the hypothalamus rely upon its receiving information concerning the body's needs from nervous and vascular sources, and that it is interlocked, both structurally and functionally, with higher regions of the nervous system. This ability to balance the body's physical needs—altering temperature, blood pressure, fluid balance, energy needs and so on—to meet changes occurring in the body is an extremely complex task. Any slight imbalance of endocrine function can result in changes which could, as an end result or side effect, cause the establishment of unwanted hair.

If the functions of the hypothalamus are studied briefly, it can clearly be seen that many of the causes of unwanted hair, both hirsutism and hypertrichosis, relate to aspects of neuroendocrinology, or endocrine function.

ENDOCRINE CONTROL

The cells of the anterior pituitary form hormone inhibiting factors which influence the production of *thyrotrophin, corticotrophin, somatotrophin, prolactin, luteinizing hormone, follicle stimulating hormone* and *melanocyte stimulating hormone*. Some of these work directly on general body tissues, while others work indirectly through the medium of a secondary endocrine organ, for example, the thyroid gland, adrenal cortex, or the gonads.

NEUROSECRETION

Neurosecretion of oxytocin and vasopressin (antidiuretic hormone ADH) affect blood pressure regulation and the fluid balance of the body.

AUTONOMIC EFFECTS

These show that many automatic functions of the body are affected by the hypothalamus, including the cardiovascular and respiratory systems and alimentary control.

TEMPERATURE REGULATION

The hypothalamus acts as a central regulating mechanism for maintaining the correct body temperature. Heat production and heat loss are produced by changes in the cutaneous blood flow—vasodilation (or expansion of the blood vessels) accompanied by sweating to lose surface heat, and constriction of surface vessels, in conjunction with shivering and 'goose pimples', diminish heat loss. The hypothalamus receives information regarding body temperature from nervous and vascular sources, and is able to instigate the correct autonomic endocrine and muscular response to maintain the correct temperature level.

FOOD AND WATER REGULATION

Controls exerted in the medial and lateral (middle and side) areas of the hypothalamus determine appetite or hunger, and also influence feelings of satiation. In this way, the body's energy needs are balanced by the correct food intake. It would seem in many overweight individuals that the satiation centre in the brain either does not work very efficiently, or can be overridden by personal taste or enjoyment of the food. Water balance, in addition to being controlled by water loss in the urine (through vasopressin), is also regulated by fluid intake dictated by thirst. The urge to drink and take in necessary fluid is controlled by the lateral zone of the hypothalamus.

REPRODUCTION AND SEXUAL BEHAVIOUR

Through its control of gonadotrophin production by the anterior pituitary, the hypothalamus controls many aspects of reproduction and sexual development and behaviour.

MAINTENANCE OF NATURAL BODY RHYTHMS

The natural pattern of sleep and wakefulness, temperature fluctuations to maintain body temperature, and biological activity to maintain cellular function and regeneration, often termed *circadian rhythms*, are controlled by the hypothalamus.

The hypothalamus appears to be the source of the many, strongly felt emotions. By its action, it causes changes in the basic drives of such things as sex, hunger and thirst, and at the same time it triggers off other systems of the body—for instance the muscular system—so giving rise to behavioural changes related to emotions such as rage, fear and pleasure. These so-called positive and negative reward centres of hypothalamic function bring into play many co-ordinated actions. This can be seen, for example, during a state of fear, when adrenaline is secreted and muscular action produces flight.

ENDOCRINE DISORDERS

Pigmentation, alterations in the texture of the skin, and changes in hair growth patterns are all important features of many endocrine disorders. It is important, therefore, for the electrologist to be aware of these disorders and their manifestations as outlined below.

Disorders of the Suprarenal Glands (Adrenal Bodies)

Lesions affecting the cortex or medulla of the suprarenal glands can result in a range of physical illnesses. These can be attributed either to an excess or a deficiency in the secretions of these parts of the gland.

UNDERSECRETION OF THE SUPRARENAL CORTEX

Addison's disease is caused by atrophy or tuberculosis of the suprarenal cortex, with consequent insufficiency of cortical secretion. The disease is characterized by muscular weakness, low blood pressure, anaemia, changes in the fluid balance of the tissue and terminal circulatory and renal failure. Brownish pigmentation (hyperpigmentation) is usually also present, involving normally pigmented areas such as the face, neck, arms and nipples, the mucous membrane of the mouth and palmar creases and scars.

EXCESSIVE SECRETION OF THE SUPRARENAL CORTEX

Excessive cortical secretion resulting from tumours or hyperplasia of the cortex may produce a number of conditions. **Cushing's syndrome** is a disease which causes the individual to become obese and suffer from excessive hairiness of the face and trunk and diabetes mellitus. In the female, excessive blood loss during the menstrual cycle may be experienced, accompanied by pain before and during the period (dysamenorrhoea). In the male, impotence can result.

Virilism

In women, excessive secretion of the androgenic hormones may result in masculinization of the secondary characters (virilism)—that is, hair grows in the male sexual pattern, on the inside thigh areas, around the umbilical area, on the breasts (chest) and in a beard formation on the face. The voice may deepen and a shrinking of the breasts can occur.

Feminism

In men, feminization may occur. This includes breast enlargement and the establishment of soft fat deposits in the female pattern.

Disorders of the Thyroid Gland

HYPERTHYROIDISM THYROTOXICOSIS (oversecretion)

Overproduction of the two thyroid hormones, *tri-iodothyronin* and *thyroxin*, leads to the condition of thyrotoxicosis, resulting in enlargement of the gland (a *goitre*). Cellular metabolism may be affected, causing weight loss, high skin temperature and increased sweating. Changes in skin pigmentation and colour can result in vitiligo and piebald skin. Hair growth is often affected, being shed in patches and changing in character.

HYPOTHROIDISM MYXOEDEMA (undersecretion)

A condition causing the skin to appear thickened, coarse and dry. It may also turn a yellowish colour due to carotinaemia being formed. Circulation will be poor and chilblains develop easily. Loss of hair is common, and the remaining hair becomes dry, brittle and scanty. The patients often become obese and slow in their movements.

Disorders of the Pituitary Gland (Hypophysis Cerebri)

ACROMEGALY

The rare disease of acromegaly is characterized by a gradual increase in the size of the hands, feet and face. Headaches and a peculiar type of blindness, brought on by the enlarging hypophysis pressing on the optic chiasma can result. This causes blindness in the upper fields of vision through atrophy of the nerve fibres, but leaves the lower fields of vision intact. Acromegaly can give rise to a thick, furrowed and wrinkled skin, with acne and comedomes. Hair growth may also be accentuated.

FRÖHLICH'S SYNDROME

A disease which causes the individual to become fat, with a smooth, pale skin. The pubic and axillary hair is absent, and the eyebrows may be scanty. The nails appear thin and without half moons (lanulas) at their base.

SIMMOND'S DISEASE

This occurs only in women, usually after childbirth. The skin appears pale and waxy, and may later become wrinkled and glossy. Axillary and eyebrow hair disappears completely.

HAIR GROWTH IN RELATION TO SEXUAL DEVELOPMENT AND THE REPRODUCTIVE CYCLE

It has been seen that hormones are chemical substances secreted by the endocrine glands directly into the bloodstream where they affect many aspects of physical development and the maintenance of normal body functions. Their effect can be seen very clearly when sexual development is considered, and throughout the different stages concerned with the reproductive cycle in women.

Even within normal hormonal levels, the incidence of unwanted hair can be high if the individual is predisposed to hypertrichosis or has a family or racial tendency towards it. If the hormonal balance is altered, however, through illness or medication which affects hormone output, then hair growth can quickly become a problem, bearing in mind that the hair follicle is an end organ of the endocrine system. Growths or cysts on the ovaries may alter the output of female hormones and allow male hormones to become more dominant, thus producing superfluous hair in areas, such as the face, where the follicles are sensitive to such a hormonal change. This type of change is not immediate, but comes as a result of androgens which are produced by the adrenals and gonads having made their presence felt over a sufficient length of time.

Hair growth that is unacceptable to an individual can develop at any stage of life as a result of alterations in hormonal output, and, whether they occur naturally or are induced through drug therapy, they quickly affect the potential growth of the follicles.

If the relationship of hormone secretion to sexual development and reproduction is studied briefly, it can be seen that many opportunities are present for unwanted hair growth to develop as a result of a small deviation from the normal hormone balance. This deviation or change may be so small as to cause no other side effects apart from unwanted hair, and may not affect the individual's capacity for normal sexual development or successful childbearing.

Adolescence

In adolescence, where the hormonal control is establishing secondary sexual characteristics, such as breast development and menstruation in the female, and beard growth and deepening of the voice in the male, a great potential exists for unwanted hair growth in the female. While the hormone levels are becoming established and fixed, a great deal of irregularity exists, which can result in skin blemishes and acne, and in women irregular menstruation and in some cases unwanted hair. Where the hormone balance is very sensitive, it can be easily disrupted by factors such as taking the Pill to avoid pregnancy, regularize erratic menstruation, or help a bad acne condition. Hair which grows in response to this stimulus in predisposed women does sometimes regress (grow less or return to normal) when the medication is stopped or a non-hormonal alternative is used. Hair growth presented for epilation in the adolescent female should only be undertaken after medical consultation to ascertain the hormonal background to the condition, and to determine whether treatment is in fact necessary or whether the condition would right itself naturally without the need for electrology.

This sensitivity to hormonal changes in the predisposed female would point to a need for the Pill being prescribed only by physicians, since only they can determine how susceptible to side effects the individual might prove to be.

After puberty, each month some follicular cells develop to form vesicular ovarian (Graafian) follicles, one of which usually matures and ruptures (ovulation). The cells of the ovaries produce oestrogenic hormones (mainly oestradiol), and the development of the Graafian follicle itself is stimulated by the gonadotrophic hormone of the hypophysis cerebri (follicle stimulating hormone—FSH). Involved in the formation of the Graafian follicle and preparation of the uterus for the fertilized ovum are initially the FSH—the luteinizing hormone (LH) and the luteotrophic hormone prolactin or lactogen (LTH)—and subsequently the ovarian hormones *progesterone* and *oestrogen* (oestradiol).

Pregnancy

If pregnancy occurs, these follicle stimulating and luteinizing hormones are known as *chorionic gonadotrophins*, and they stimulate the corpus luteum of menstruation to increase in size and prolong its activity. These ovarian hormones are necessary to achieve conception and a successful pregnancy, while the placenta plays an important role as an endocrine organ in sustaining the unborn child until birth. Some women require additional hormone drug medication to maintain the pregnancy and prevent miscarriage, or in cases of subfertility (low fertility) to achieve conception at all (fertility drugs). In both instances, hair growth can result from the hormone medication. It appears after a period of time has elapsed, usually after the birth, when the effect of the gonadotrophic hormones has built up and made its presence felt in the body systems. This hair growth manifests itself as an increased level and density of normal facial hair, with the follicles stimulated to greater activity and acquiring an increased blood supply by growing deeper into the dermis. Because of the endocrine stimulation involved, these hairs can be extremely difficult to remove, and have an abnormal regrowth potential. It is better, therefore, to work for extreme accuracy in the epilation removals, rather than speed of removal.

The *lactogenic hormone* (LTH), or mammotrophin, stimulates the mammary glands in preparation for breast-feeding, and controls the secretion of milk from the milk ducts of the breasts.

Thus, it is seen that ovarian hormones are involved in the preparation of the body for pregnancy, the formation of the ovarian follicle, ovulation, and sustaining the pregnancy. The reproductive cycle is, therefore, intrinsically linked with the endocrine system and falls entirely under its control through the gonadotrophic hormones. Many opportunities present themselves for hormonal imbalance, either naturally or as a result of the administration of hormone therapy to maintain the health of the mother or child.

In some cases, simply the increased levels of ovarian hormones circulating in the bloodstream during pregnancy is sufficient to trigger increased hair growth, and this problem worsens with subsequent pregnancies, especially if they are closely spaced.

Menopause

As the menopause, or 'change of life', approaches, the reproductive role of the body is over and the female hormones lose their dominance or controlling power over the male hormone, *testosterone.* These, then, are able to obtain an influence over the body systems and cause changes to occur such as loss of menstruation, shrinking of the breast tissue, and, in many cases, unwanted hair growth on the upper lip and chin, and, in some cases the throat. This occurrence is so common in middle-aged women that it cannot be classed as an abnormality, rather it should be considered as an annoying aspect of the ageing process for those predisposed to the problem. Alongside unwanted hair growth often come pigmentation problems—brown spots, the formation of fibrous lumps, etc. Many of these conditions, like superfluous hair, can be successfully treated, and the client should be encouraged to deal with them to maintain a youthful appearance.

Women who have a partial or total hysterectomy may suffer from lack of secretion of the ovarian hormones, oestrogen and progesterone. In young women, an attempt is often made to retain the ovaries (partial hysterectomy) in order to allow normal ovarian secretion to continue so as to maintain a normal, healthy life. Lack of ovarian hormonal secretion may cause tiredness, lack of sexual drive, and at the same time affects the fragility of bone tissues, thus making the individual more susceptible to fractures. Some women are given hormone replacement therapy (HRT) to replace those hormones lost through removal of the womb and ovaries. Opinion differs as to the relative advantages and dangers of hormone replacement therapy, because in the normal way ovarian secretion output reduces naturally with age. With HRT, however, an artificially high level of hormones is maintained in the body beyond the age at which the menopause would occur if the womb and ovaries were intact.

With surgical removal of the ovaries, removal of one ovary through disease, or removal of a cyst on an ovary, an imbalance of ovarian hormones is inevitable, even if oestrogen medication is given to redress the balance. Both the actual condition and the controlling drug medication can result in the establishment of superfluous hair. In the same way, both the hysterectomy and the balancing and compensatory hormone replacement therapy can be the direct cause of unwanted hair growth.

When all the possibilities for unwanted hair linked with the reproductive cycle are considered, the need for medical referral to guide the electrologist becomes very evident.

Chapter 6

Clinical Pathology. Common Skin Disorders

The electrologist must have a sound, basic knowledge of the common skin disorders which may be encountered in the course of her work. As most clients consult the electrologist directly, rather than being referred by a doctor, there is a risk that the individual may be suffering from a skin complaint which is infectious or for which epilation is contra-indicated (prohibited). As has already been observed, a high standard of clinic hygiene must be maintained in order to prevent infection occurring as a result of treatment, and also special sterilization procedures undertaken to eliminate the risk of cross-infection taking place where skin complaints are present. Some skin disorders limit or alter treatment, but do not prevent its application—for example, diabetes and psoriasis—while others require special treatment planning to achieve successful results—for example, skins prone to eczema or dermatitis reactions require variable spacing of the probes and extended periods between treatments to promote skin healing. So, *recognition* of skin disorders, as well as some knowledge of their cause and the risks of contagion, are essential information to the operator.

The electrologist may also be consulted regarding the removal of hairs from moles. It is most important in such a case that the operator is fully cognisant of all the facts relating to the moles, and able to determine immediately whether she may treat the patient or whether medical referral should be advised. These more advanced aspects of electrology including treatment of surface capillaries (broken veins), spider naevi, blood spots, small fibrous growths, etc., come under the general description of *minor cosmetic electrology*, and are dealt with in Chapter 7. These are areas of treatment which may be advanced to when basic experience has been expanded, together with a thorough knowledge of the skin and its reactions to treatment. For, in these cases, it is not simply a knowledge of how to perform the task that is required, but rather the ability to estimate how the skin will react and how it will stand up to the diathermy application. This is the deciding factor in determining whether or not to perform minor cosmetic electrology, and because skins are so diverse in their reactions, it is a difficult and responsible decision. Many electrologists, therefore, prefer to concentrate on hair removal, and do not undertake any work in this area.

The more that is known about the skin and its disorders (blemishes, pigmentation problems, fibrous growths and alterations through illness), the more confidence the operator will have in her work. Furthermore, understanding the cause of the condition will give the electrologist an insight into the form the disorder will take and its likely development—vital points when planning long-term programmes of treatment.

The best way to approach the problem of skin disorders is to seek medical approval for the treatment of any condition which seems suspect and where the cause of the problem is unknown. This safeguards both the client and the operator. Since the electrologist is not medically qualified, it is not within her field of reference to diagnose skin conditions. Rather, it is her task to see that her client receives only the most suitable treatment, and to ensure that, where epilation would prolong or aggravate a skin complaint, it is not offered.

DERMATOLOGICAL TERMS IN USE

Erythema—redness of the skin.

Macule—a mark or discolouration of the skin, which can be seen but not felt.

Wheal—the fully developed wheal is red, white at the centre, raised above the surface, and has a superficial lumpy feel. It may vary in size from a centimetre in diameter to a plaque many centimetres in surface area.

Papule—a firm, raised lump. It does not contain fluid, may be vascular in appearance and varies in size from a pinhead to half a centimetre.

Vesicle—a small elevation in the skin containing fluid.

Bulla—a larger blister.

Pustule—a pustule is a lesion which commences as a papule and becomes purulent in the centre (containing pus). Pustules develop at the mouths of hair follicles, appearing as inflamed red areas, with central cores of pus, from which hairs may project.

Pigmentation—skin colour; hyperpigmentation, increased colour, brown or red coloration.

Primary lesions—vesicles, pustules and weals.

Secondary lesions—ulcers, scales, crusts and scars.

Erythema

Erythema is a diffused, deep pink or red flush of the skin, produced by an increase in the skin temperature. The redness of the skin disappears on pressure. There are many causes of erythema (or skin reddening): it may precede an illness, if it is generalized, or be a result of injury or trauma, if localized. Erythema can be associated with an allergic reaction to foods, drugs, plants, etc., or it may be a simple irritant reaction to wool or clothing, or rough textured blankets. Erythema is associated with sunburn, windburn, overexposure to cold weather, skin chapping and any condition where the skin is subjected to injury. Extremely high skin temperature, sweating, etc., will cause erythema; sometimes it precedes a heat rash, urticaria (hives) or contact dermatitis. Many infectious diseases are preceded by erythema rashes, for example, measles, scarlatina and rubella. If a client is hot and flushed, it may simply indicate that she feels unwell and is perhaps heading for influenza or a nasty cold. On the other hand, it may relate to a number of other conditions, and the operator must, therefore, be aware of all the implications.

ERYTHEMA FOLLOWING EPILATION TREATMENT

Erythema occurs after epilation applications as a direct result of the skin trauma experienced, and is often present in association with inflammation and oedema (swelling) of the area. The skin tissues react to the cautery produced by the diathermy current, which coagulates the base of the follicle and hair root. The skin's normal defence mechanisms against bacteria are brought into action, and the white blood cells (leucocytes) start off the healing process, causing increased skin temperature and activity in the damaged area.

Some individuals experience severe erythema reaction to epilation, and also suffer from swelling, scabbing and general soreness of the treatment area for several days. This points to a need to adapt the treatment application and use every technique to reduce the skin reaction: these may include the use of insulated needles, additional spacing of the probes, low current strength and well-spaced treatment intervals. The importance of excellent, skin soothing lotions during treatment can be clearly seen where erythema reaction is concerned. If a severe reaction can be prevented, the other side effects of epilation are at least reduced, if not entirely removed, and the skin's recovery is much enhanced, thus allowing treatment to progress at an effective pace, without causing skin dehydration, scarring or pitting.

Every endeavour must be made either to *avoid* creating a severe erythema reaction by excellent practical technique, or to *reduce* the reaction by careful precare, aftercare and home-care measures.

LIST OF COMMON SKIN DISORDERS

Fibroma—non-malignant, fibrous growth of skin.

Verruca—infectious wart.

Naevus—vascular and pigmented birthmark (plural: **naevi**).

Angioma—vascular tumour.

Haemangioma—vascular naevus (alternative name for the commonest type of naevus).

Papilloma—mole (alternative name).

Dermatitis—inflammation and irritation of the skin (non-infectious).

Contact dermatitis—non-infectious inflammation of the skin due to contact with external agents.

Acne vulgaris—infection of the hair follicle involving excessive oil secretion. A non-infectious condition, but requiring strict hygienic precautions in the clinic if secondary infection is present.

Seborrhoea—excessive secretion of the sebaceous glands.

Sebaceous cyst—an overgrowth of epidermal tissue which traps sebaceous matter into a cyst-like formation.

Acne rosacea—non-infectious condition of nervous origin affecting the nose and cheeks, with skin erythema and seborrhoea.

Eczema—irritation and overproliferation of the skin (increased and excessive shedding).

Asteatosis—a breakdown in sebaceous secretion, causing extreme dryness of skin.

Lichen planus—small, shiny, pink or purple papules, the size of a pinhead, normally occurring in multiple form, affecting the arms and legs.

Senile bruising, purpura—causes reddish-black pigmentation in old age.

Chloasma—a harmless pigmentation condition associated with pregnancy.

Lentigo—a pigmentation condition rather like freckles but unaffected by sunlight.

Vitiligo, leucoderma—pigmentation disorder, in which there are white patches or loss of pigmentation.

Albinism—total absence of pigment in the tissues.

Urticaria (hives)—allergic reaction to food, drugs, etc., which forms a red, itchy rash. It can also be a heat reaction.

Allergic reaction—abnormal response to a specific substance; created by the formation of antibodies in the blood following previous exposure to the substance.

Boil, carbuncle—result of inflammation of hair follicles due to staphylococcal infection, and denotes lowered resistance to infection.

Psoriasis—non-infectious condition of nervous origin causing patches of oval, red skin surrounded by silvery scales.

Impetigo—highly infectious, red rash, beginning with blisters and followed by pus and crusting of the skin. A condition associated with dirt and poor living conditions.

Scabies—infectious condition of parasitic origin, caused by tiny mites which burrow under the skin in zigzag lines culminating in red blisters. Very itchy and considered a condition associated with dirty living situations.

Herpes simplex (cold sore)—virus infection affecting the mouth.

Herpes zoster (shingles)—highly infectious condition which starts on the bridge of the nose, runs under the eye and over the forehead, affecting the nerves of the head.

Warts—virus infection of the skin, highly infectious.

Ringworm—fungus infection of the skin and scalp. The condition has many forms and is infectious.

Tinea pedis (athlete's foot)—highly infectious, fungus infection affecting the clefts between the toes.

Hyperidrosis—a condition of excessive perspiration.

Bromidrosis—excessive perspiration and bad body odour.

DISORDERS OF THE FOLLICLE AND SEBACEOUS GLAND

Acne Vulgaris

Acne vulgaris is an inflammation of the sebaceous gland which lies just beneath the surface of the skin, causing pimples, blackheads, papules, pustules, and sometimes infected cysts and scarring. The skin appears greasy and has a dull, sallow colour. It is most commonly found in adolescents, and it may involve the entire face, chest and shoulder girdle, or be confined in any one of these areas. Seborrhoea is present, resulting in the formation of comedones of varying intensities depending on the influence of the endocrine glands on the sebaceous secretion. The dark colour of the blackhead is due to the development of sulphides in the keratinized cells of the surface blockage. Not all follicles become blocked, but removal of surface oiliness and skin blockage reduces the possibility of the acne condition spreading. A staphylococcal infection sometimes produces a secondary infection, with inflammation and pustules forming around the horny blackhead. The infection may spread to involve the sebaceous gland, and then a deep-seated pustular condition becomes established. Many acne eruptions leave disfiguring scars, and so must be dealt with medically if secondary infection is present. If medical agreement is given, therapy treatment can be applied to good effect to control the condition and improve its management.

Seborrhoea

Seborrhoea is caused by overactivity of the sebaceous glands, secretion, an excess of sebum and abnormal oiliness of the skin's surface. The situation and density of the sebaceous glands in the scalp, face, centre of the chest and back cause the seborrhoea to be most evident in these areas. During puberty, the activity of the glands is increased as a result of hormonal changes, and the sebaceous gland ducts and hair follicles become enlarged, the skin becomes coarser and open pores are evident. The excessive, oily secretion blocks the outward flow of sebum to the surface, and it becomes lodged in the follicle and sebaceous duct. The retained sebum increases in volume, and the external area hardens and becomes overlaid with epidermal cells to form a comedone (blackhead). Seborrhoea is the basis of several skin diseases, particularly acne vulgaris.

Acne Rosacea

Acne rosacea, like acne vulgaris, is an eruption which affects the face, and is associated with seborrhoea. The cutaneous vessels of the nose and cheeks are the most affected, giving a red, flushed appearance, particularly after the intake of food, or due to a change in temperature. The disease may be long-standing, and is disfiguring as the skin surface becomes lumpy and thickened with papules and pustules. Rosacea is sometimes confused with acne vulgaris, due to its location, but rosacea seldom appears before the age of 30, while acne vulgaris has usually regressed by that age.

Sebaceous Cyst (Steatoma)

A sebaceous cyst (also known as a wen) becomes blocked by an overgrowth of surface skin tissue and the sebum becomes encapsulated within the fibrous casing. The cyst has no opening to the skin's surface, but can be excised by a cosmetic surgeon very effectively, leaving little trace. Some individuals seem very prone to cysts, and may have them in multiple formation. Although treatment of them is not a part of the electrologist's work, if they are present in the treatment area they will affect the epilation application.

Asteatosis

This is a condition in which the sebaceous system is considered to have broken down. No sebum is secreted, causing the skin to be extremely dry and susceptible to chapping, scaling and splitting. It responds to medical treatment.

SKIN DISEASES OF NERVOUS ORIGIN

Herpes Simplex (Cold Sore)

An inflammation of the skin is accompanied by the formation of clusters of small blisters around the mouth and nostril areas, brought on by an acute virus infection. The eruption begins as an itchy patch of erythema, which develops into weeping vesicles if scratched. Herpes simplex is a recurring disease, which lasts for a few days, usually leaving no trace. The area should be left alone, and any electrology treatment postponed until the condition has cleared.

Eczema (Dermatitis)

This skin condition begins as an itching, red area, with pinhead-sized vesicles, and progresses to a scaly, dry patchiness, or continued vesicle formation and weeping. These symptoms may occur on any part of the body and at any time of life.

Eczema is a tissue reaction involving the epidermis and upper layers of the dermis, caused by:
(1) External contact with a substance to which the skin is allergic (exogenous);
(2) Internal stimulus via the bloodstream (endogenous).

Eczema can also develop on the lower part of the legs when varicose veins are present. The skin takes on a shiny, glazed appearance, with a congestion of the blood supply giving a bluish, red colour, and evident split capillaries. The condition could develop into a varicose ulcer, and as the skin cracks easily due to its impaired blood supply, no treatment must be attempted.

Psoriasis

Psoriasis can affect the entire body and facial areas, but is often seen on the limbs, especially on the knees and elbows. The lesions of psoriasis begin as dull, red papules, the size of pinheads, and they develop into plaques which are bright red in colour, with sharply defined margins. The patches of psoriasis may have flaky, silvery-white scales overlying the surface, which give the condition a distinct appearance. The cause of the condition is not known, but it does appear to be a recurring complaint, and in some cases may be present in small areas most of an individual's life.

Psoriasis may attack the nail fold, or the nail bed, and causes pitting of the nail plate and a build up of cells under the free edge.

All psoriasis conditions of the skin and nails require medical attention, although a small proportion of clients may have small areas which appear at times of stress and which may not prohibit treatment as long as the area involved is completely avoided and the client's doctor is in agreement with the treatment being undertaken.

PIGMENTATION ABNORMALITIES
Naevi (Vascular and Pigmented Birthmarks)

SPIDER NAEVUS (TELANGIECTATIC ANGIOMA)

The spider naevus consists of a central dilated vessel, with smaller capillaries radiating from it like the legs of a spider. It is often called a *broken vein*, and may be found in isolation or in a general area of vascular skin such as the cheeks. The spider naevus usually develops in adult life, and is commonly found on the face, particularly on the upper cheek and eye areas.

PORT WINE STAIN (CAPILLARY ANGIOMA)

The port wine stain consists of a large area of dilated capillaries, resulting in a skin colour ranging from pink to dark red, which presents a vivid contrast with the surrounding skin. The stain is commonly found on the face and, as the skin texture is usually normal, application of cosmetic masking camouflage is very successful in alleviating embarrassment and distress. The port wine stain does not usually regress, and the treatment for it is limited.

STRAWBERRY MARK
(SUPERFICIAL CAVERNOUS
ANGIOMA)

A brightly pigmented skin area, seen at birth or developing soon afterwards, which usually disappears before adult life.

PIGMENTED NAEVI

Pigmented naevi may occur on any part of the body, and are often found on the neck and face, sometimes associated with strong hair growth (*pigmented hairy naevi*). They vary in size from a pinhead to several centimetres in diameter and in only very rare cases may be extremely large. The pigmentation present may vary from light brown to very dark or black. Pigmented naevi, with the exception of the coal black variety, are classed as benign tumours, and their removal is usually for cosmetic reasons.

Papillomas (Moles)

Moles are a form of pigmented naevi and are a common occurrence on the face and body. They present several different forms, varying in size, colour and vascular appearance. Flat colourless moles are termed 'sessile', while those which are raised above the surface, attached by a stalk, are said to be 'pedunculated'. All raised and pigmented moles require medical approval before electrology treatment is given, or they can be removed surgically if they cause distress.

Flat Pigmented Mole
Flat moles are normally brownish-black in colour, with sharp margins, and have the same feel as normal skin.

These may be found to a greater or lesser extent on every individual. The essential feature is the presence of melanin in localized places in the connective tissue cells of the cutis. A pigmented naevus is a benign tumour, although melanin, normally an ingredient of the epidermis, is not an epithelial cell. Therefore, the flat pigmented naevus can be classed with pigmentary disorders rather than with tumours. For this reason, moles are covered by a wide variety of descriptions; sometimes they are called moles or tumours, naevi or fibroma, as they may fit into any or several of these classifications. Occasionally, a pigmented mole may undergo a malignant change and skin cancer may arise from it, and, although this is a rare occurrence, it is an important point to remember in epilation and removal of hairs from moles. Any interference with a mole could cause this change to occur, and hence medical approval must be sought prior to treatment.

Raised Pigmented Mole

This is a naevus in which connective tissue as well as pigment is hypertrophied (built up or overdeveloped), and which is really a fibroma. The mole may be harder or softer than the surrounding tissues, and vary in colour from deep brown to normal skin colour. It can be felt as a raised area above the surrounding skin, and be single or multiple in formation. These skin growths can be removed surgically if they cause embarrassment, and do not come within the work of the electrologist unless under direct medical supervision in the hospital situation.

Hairy Mole (Naevus Pilosus)

Hairy moles may be raised or flat, and have strong hairs growing from them. These moles are usually pigmented, brownish in colour, and can be really large and disfiguring. The hairs growing from moles can be epilated with medical approval. They are normally very deeply placed, requiring very accurate probing to reach the hair root. The deepest point of the pigment is normally at the base of the hairs, and when the hairs are removed the mole decreases in colour intensity and size (if it is a small growth).

In older people, pigmented moles can occasionally begin to enlarge suddenly, or the Malpighian layer in them may begin to proliferate; the colour of the mole fades, it becomes wart-like, and requires medical attention. These are termed *naevi seniles*, and are a pre-cancerous condition of the skin.

Any pigmented mole which has changed rapidly in size or colour should receive medical attention, as it could indicate a cancerous condition elsewhere in the body. Black moles may be a secondary sign of a primary cancer in the body, and must *not* be treated in any way.

Pigmentation Abnormalities

CHLOASMA

This pigmentation condition consists of harmless, light-brown patches of irregular size and shape on the skin. It is most frequently associated with pregnancy, involving the upper cheeks, nose and occasionally the forehead areas of the face. The discoloration usually disappears spontaneously with the termination of the pregnancy, but if it persists, ordinary desquamation therapy methods will affect a cure.

VITILIGO

Here there is complete loss of colour in the skin and hairs in well-defined areas of the body, face and limbs. It begins as small patches which may converge to form fairly large areas. The skin around the patches sometimes appears hyperpigmented, and the condition is most obvious on darker-skinned individuals. The basal cells are no longer able to manufacture melanin, and so the areas must be protected from ultraviolet exposure, or the skin will become irritated. Cosmetic camouflage can be used to disguise prominent areas on the face, neck or hands which cause anxiety or embarrassment to the client.

FRECKLES (EPHELIDES)

Ephelides are small pigmented areas of skin, which become more evident on exposure to sunlight and are found in greatest abundance on the face, arms and legs. Fair-skinned individuals suffer most from the condition, which can be cosmetically disfiguring, especially on red-haired women, where the freckles join up to form large patches. The intensity of the colour can be reduced by bleaching creams and peeling pastes, but will reappear on exposure to sunlight.

LENTIGO

These darker areas of pigmentation appear more distinct than freckles and have a slightly raised appearance and more scattered distribution. They do not increase in colour density or number on exposure to sunlight.

Fungus Infections

RINGWORM

Ringworm infections account for a large part of all skin infections likely to need medical help for their cure. There are three main genera of ringworm:
(1) Microsporon;
(2) Trichophyton (endothrix and ectothrix);
(3) Epidermophyton.
However, there are many species, some of which will be considered.
Ringworm is a fungus infection and comes within the dermatophytes group of fungi which produce superficial infection (termed dermatomy-

cosis) of the skin, hair and nails. The well-known names *ringworm* and *tinea* do not, unfortunately, cover all varieties of fungus infection, as there are many other types of fungus involved apart from these.

Microsporon Ringworm

Within the ringworm group the microsporon fungus affects the surface of the skin and grows within the hair shaft bringing about the condition known as *tinea capitis* (ringworm of the scalp). The vast majority of cases are due to the microsporon audouini (a variety peculiar to the human species) or microsporon canis (animal origin). Tinea capitis manifests itself as round scaly patches, with broken hairs, giving a bald appearance. The condition is most common in children, but does affect adults.

Trichophyton Ringworm

Bald patches on the scalp where the hairs assume a dot-like appearance may be due to the trichophyton fungus, though this is much less common. The 'black dot' ringworm is in fact a condition where only the hairs are attacked: they then break off at the surface showing a pigmented stump. The species involved is the trichophyton endothrix, mostly of human origin.

Where the condition is more inflammatory and the patches are more scaly and clearly defined, the fungus may be the trichophyton ectothrix; this is of animal origin, coming mainly from horses, cattle, cats and dogs. This uncommon condition often leaves bald patches after treatment is completed (alopecia), and is, therefore, extremely disfiguring.

Tinea Barbae

Ringworm of the beard is caused by the endothrix and ectothrix trichophytons, taking superficial or deep forms depending on severity. The superficial type shows scaly patches, with partial hair loss in the affected places. The hairs are brittle, and show enlarged, white bulbous roots on removal. Alopecia can result in the affected areas, making this an extremely disfiguring, but uncommon, problem. The deep form of the condition produces deep pustules and nodules, in addition to the hair loss, and is mainly found affecting the lower cheeks and neck. The condition may be localized along the jawline, and is complicated by the process of shaving, which must normally be discontinued in the affected areas.

Tinea Circinata

Ringworm of the skin is caused by various forms of trichophyton and microsporon and is described as *tinea circinata*. The lesions are ringed, single or multiple, and vary in severity, from mild scaling to inflamed itching areas. The primary lesion is a small, red macule which spreads outwards as it heals in the centre. The ringed appearance is often distinctive. Most common in children, the patches affect the face, shoulders and neck areas most frequently.

Epidermophyton Ringworm

The epidermophyton genus of ringworm is a fungus closely related to the trichophyton variety, but it does not affect the hair, only the skin, hence the name *epidermophyton*, an epidermal fungus. The conditions *tinea cruris, tinea pedis* and *tinea unguium* may all be traced to this genus through different species.

Tinea Cruris

This is an acute eruption on the groin and inside thigh area, and is more common in males. The epidermophyton inguinal (floccosum) form is the most common cause, but occasionally it can be traced to forms of trichophyton. The scaly lesions often have the appearance of eczema, and are extremely irritating.

Tinea Pedis (Athlete's Foot)

This is mainly caused by the epidermophyton inguinal (floccosum) form and involves the toes and the sole of the foot. The lesion on the foot may be the primary one, and elsewhere on the body may be seen other eruptions of a fungus type. Tinea pedis is extremely common, and infectious, but is fairly easy to control. The skin between the toes assumes a sodden appearance, and when rubbed off shows deep splits in the skin and a raw, reddened area.

Tinea Unguium

Ringworm of the nails, can be caused by the trichophyton or epidermophyton types, but it may have other causes. The nails are attacked from either the free edge or from the nail fold, and assume a distorted, horny appearance. The nail plate becomes discoloured, rough, opaque and very disfigured. In most cases, the nails of the feet will be affected prior to the hands becoming involved.

Common Warts (Verruca Vulgaris)

These are firm papules with a rough horny surface which range in size from less than a millimetre to over a centimetre in diameter. Warts are caused by a virus infection and can be acquired by contact with another person suffering from the condition, as they are highly contagious. Common warts occur most frequently on the hands, but can be found in all areas of the face and body. The warts are often dark in colour, and form groups on the backs of the hands, around the nail fold and sometimes under the nail. They often have a multiple formation, and, after varying periods of time, tend to disappear spontaneously.

Flat Warts (Verruca Plana)

These appear as smooth, pearly, epidermal elevations, about the size of pinheads, usually found in groups, and most frequently situated on the face and hands.

All kinds of warts can be removed surgically, or with diathermy, and plantar warts often respond to treatment which excludes the air, for example, airtight plasters. Many warts have been seen to disappear with simple psychotherapy techniques.

Verruca Plantaris

These are warts which are found on the soles of the feet. They become flattened by pressure, so that they do not project beyond the surface. They may be single or multiple, and usually become painful at some stage of their development, and they should be attended to as early as possible in order to avoid spreading the condition, or causing unnecessary discomfort.

ALLERGIC SKIN CONDITIONS

An allergic reaction is seen as an abnormal response to a specific substance, brought about by antibodies in the blood which have been formed after a previous exposure to the substance concerned. There are many forms of allergy which appear as an urticaria or eczematous dermatitis reaction, although it should be remembered that these conditions may also be due to other causes. The allergic reaction may be due to *ingestion* of a foreign protein, *inhalation* as in hay fever, or *contact* with a sensitizing agent. Detecting the underlying cause of an allergic reaction is a medical responsibility, and should not be attempted by the electrologist. However, due to the complex nature of allergic reactions in clients, it is necessary for the electrologist to be cautious in her applications, particularly on any individual who has a history of previous allergy.

On many occasions, what appears to be a mild allergic reaction, may in fact be a primary irritation caused by the application of an unsuitable substance. Primary irritants, such as caustic preparations, highly perfumed creams, and alcohol-based lotions should be avoided, and hypo-allergenic or neutral products used.

The true allergy is a specific type of reaction, and is said to be a *specific, acquired, altered capacity to react*. It usually follows the same pattern: exposure to the substance or item, a period of time elapsing in which the blood forms antibodies, and lastly, a reapplication or re-exposure to the sensitizer causing an allergic reaction.

Urticaria (hives)

Urticaria is an acute or chronic allergic reaction in the form of an elevation of the skin to red weals, ranging in size from the size of a dot to a few centimetres in diameter, forming itchy patches. The distribution of the eruption may be local or widespread, and individual lesions usually subside within a few hours. Urticaria may be caused by an allergic reaction from either internal or external sources. The most common cause is the introduction of a foreign protein, which causes the tissue cells to release histamine, bringing about the dilatation of surface blood vessels and the creation of itchy, swollen patches. The condition usually corrects itself, but in some extreme cases medical advice is needed to determine the cause of the attack and eliminate it.

SKIN IMPERFECTIONS

Skin Tags

A common, fibrous skin condition, associated with ageing and most frequently found on the neck (especially on the sides of the neck, where they form a tear drop arrangement) and major flexures of the middle-aged and elderly. The tags form a single or multiple distribution, and they are of a soft, pedunculated form, being made up of loose fibrous tissue. The colour may be unchanged, but is often hyperpigmented, making them more obvious. The stalks of the tags can be treated successfully with diathermy coagulation by a skilled electrologist, trained in minor cosmetic surgery, once medical approval has been granted.

Whiteheads (Milia)

A whitehead is formed when sebum becomes trapped in a blind duct, which has no surface opening. The condition is most common on dry skin, and the milia appear frequently on the orbicularis oculi muscle area (that is around the eyes) and between the brows. Milia can form after injury, such as sunburn, on the face or shoulders, and are sometimes widespread in their location. Whiteheads which have been recently formed can disappear spontaneously after a period of regular massage treatment, appearing to be reabsorbed by the body. Well-established milia have to be pierced, with a sterile probe or by diathermy, to create an opening to the surface to release the contents. The whiteheads appear as pearly, rounded lumps under the skin, or raised above it, depending on their size. When the skin is stretched, the milia become more obvious and white in colour. The delicate nature of their location and the risk of infection require an experienced approach to the removal in order to prevent discomfort. Strict attention must be given to personal and salon hygiene, and to the aftercare advice to the client.

Split Capillaries

Dilated capillaries on a fine skin texture assume a general, vascular appearance, often affecting large areas of the face. The skin responds fiercely to stimulation, and permanent, dilated vessels are apparent, particularly on the upper cheeks and nose. The fineness of the skin and its general sensitivity give guidance as to the probability of split capillary formation. Ruptured blood vessels assume a line-like appearance in surface tissues, and can become bulbous and blue in colour due to the congestion of vascular circulation in the area.

Treatment success varies, depending on the location, intensity and establishment of the condition, but can be very satisfactory in certain cases. Early stages of capillary damage can be arrested by cosmetic treatments and additional protective measures including avoidance of exposure to ultraviolet rays. Ruptured or dilated vessels can only be reduced by diathermy or chemical coagulation methods. These should be applied with caution and special attention paid to the client's general skin condition. Removal of minor skin blemishes by diathermy is a specialized field of epilation, which requires additional training and experience in order to ensure success.

Rodent Ulcer (Basal Cell Carcinoma)

The ulcer looks initially like a red, unhealthy patch of skin with a slightly raised edge, which itches and irritates, but is not painful. The sore may weep and have pearly nodules around its margins. The position on the face, normally on a line between the corner of the eye and the nostril, gives guidance as to the nature of the condition. The most common site, however, is on the side of the nose, where, if left untreated, it would attack the bone tissue, hence the common name, *rodent ulcer*. The ulcer can be a skin cancer (basal cell carcinoma), and in older women is not a rare condition, so it should be watched for in electrology practice. If medically treated in its early stages (normally excised surgically), the condition can be resolved before it causes serious problems.

Chapter 7

Advanced Techniques: Minor Cosmetic Electrology

For those electrologists who wish to progress beyond simply the removal of unwanted hairs, the next stage is to venture into the realm of minor cosmetic surgery. Here, they will have the opportunity to expand their practice to include the treatment of minor skin imperfections, such as small fibrous growths (either flat or raised from the skin), thread veins (broken veins or dilated capillaries), spider naevi or blood spots, as well as the removal of hairs growing in sensitive or difficult locations, which frequently cause client distress, and those where medical approval must be sought before treatment can be given, such as hairs growing from moles or those growing on the breasts.

Such treatment calls for considerable skill and experience, and not every electrologist will wish to undertake such work, nor in fact have the ability to do so. It requires a singular capacity to bear the trauma and discomfort experienced by clients and the utmost concentration to effect the treatment successfully.

For this reason, advanced work of this kind is charged on a different basis from ordinary hair removal and must be timed differently. Despite this, however, the techniques used to accomplish many of these advanced applications are to a large extent the same as those used for basic hair removal: what does differ is the *knowledge* required to achieve a good result. This knowledge will be the basis for deciding the manner of the applications, the length of the sessions, the skin's capacity for treatment, the spacing of the applications and the timing of rest periods between treatments to allow both the skin and client to recover. This knowledge will perhaps more importantly indicate when treatment *should not be applied*—where it is contra-indicated or where the client will receive no benefit from the applications.

Possibly the most difficult aspect of advanced work is knowing when skin will not stand up to treatment (perhaps due to previous damage, as is often the case when treating dilated capillaries) or when it can be further damaged by the application rather than improved in appearance. This knowledge comes only from experience and observation of the skin under many different treatment situations, and advanced work should not be attempted until the operator is fully confident in her basic electrology techniques.

TREATMENT OF EYEBROW HAIRS

The probing technique called for here simply requires excellent handling abilities, and a delicate touch to accomplish a good result. Owing to the extreme sensitivity of the area and the proximity of the optic nerves, great care must be taken to probe the follicles *accurately* and *gently* and to use the minimum diathermy current necessary to accomplish the hair destruction.

If the eyebrows are heavy and generally unsightly and the client is of a hirsute appearance overall, a reshaping plan should be worked out at the start of the treatment to improve the eyebrows in stages so that they will not appear uneven at any time. In many instances of heavy brows, the hairs will not have been previously removed by plucking or other temporary removal methods, and so are free from follicle distortion and, therefore, ideal for epilation.

Firstly, the electrologist should discuss with the client the desired shape and thickness of the brows, and then explain the normal method by which this can be accomplished. This will give the client some idea of how long the sequence may take, and also provide an opportunity to indicate the need for her co-operation on home-care measures (not plucking the brows in between treatments, for example).

The hair removal should progress according to the plan, with the different areas of the brows being treated equally to keep the brows balanced. The hairs between the brows can be removed progressively, a little at a time to allow the skin to recover, and hairs under the brows removed with well-spaced applications, using the desired shape as a guide. Most clients are simply concerned with reducing the overall size of the eyebrow and will happily leave the new shape to the operator. A refined version of the original shape is a good shape to aim for while initial removal is taking place. The final shaping—angles of the ends of the brows, the angle of the brow arch, etc.—can be left until the eyebrow epilation is closer to the conclusion of the sequence.

Application

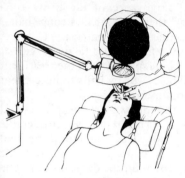

WORKING POSITION FOR
BROW EPILATION

The client should be positioned with her head well back or flat, and the operator should normally stand, as this gives greater freedom of movement to reach the difficult positioning angles required. However, if the operator prefers to sit, the client can be tipped well back on the reclining couch, provided she feels comfortable in that position, so that a flat treatment area is presented to the operator.

The probes **between the brows** are very upright, and are normally fairly shallow, although naturally this depends on the overall diameter of the hairs. The hirsute individual can have excessively strong hairs in the brows, and may need some of the long, horny hairs removed from the mass of the brow itself.

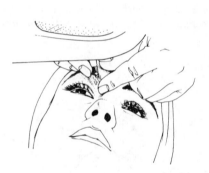

WORKING POSITION FOR
BROW EPILATION—CLOSE UP

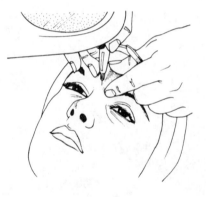

MID-BROW EPILATION

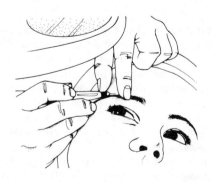

SIDE-BROW EPILATION

SIDE-BROW EPILATION—TURNED TO SIDE

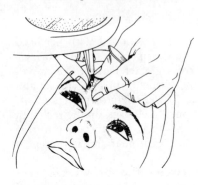

**REMOVING LARGE HAIRS
FROM THE EYEBROW MASS**

Removal of these strong hairs can reduce the size and straggly appearance of the brow considerably, but, as they are such strong hairs, requiring considerable current intensity to effect their removal, only a few should be dealt with at any one time, well interspersed with the treatment of mid-, side- and below-brow hairs to keep client discomfort to a minimum.

Probes **below the brows** are steeply angled into the skin tissue. This requires considerable concentration and skill. The skin should be held firmly over the brow bone, and care should be taken not to press down on the eyeball itself. The skin here is very fine and soft in texture, making hairs difficult to probe, and, therefore, very fine diameter needles are used to gain entry to the follicle. The operator must be acutely aware of when she has reached the base of each follicle, since incorrectly placed or excessive use of current in this area can result in a bad reaction. Bruising, blood spotting, pigmentation patches, or loss of skin colour can result from careless treatment in this area, *so it really is work of an advanced nature, and not to be attempted until technique is well developed.*

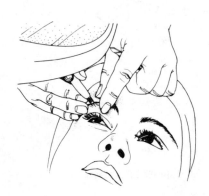

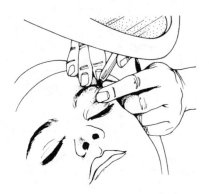

BELOW-BROW EPILATION—3 DIFFERENT ANGLES

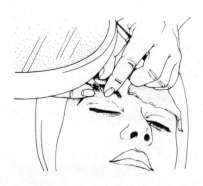

Two or three weeks should be allowed between appointments if most areas of the brow are being treated, and the client must be persuaded not to interfere with the brow during the course of the treatment programme. To do so hinders the healing process and delays the progress of the work. Furthermore, it will prevent those hairs from being treated and present a false picture of the progress achieved.

As, once treated, hairs may not regrow, care must be taken to remove only those hairs not needed to form the final brow shape. Unlike plucking, where mistakes can be erased by regrowth of the hairs, in epilation this is not the case. Operators should, therefore, keep a constant check on their work, continually assessing both brows for balance and shape.

It can take many months to accomplish a refined shape on very heavy brows, but as they are improving in appearance all the time, clients are normally well pleased with the progress. Normal precare and aftercare measures are needed with brow hair removal, and use of tinted, medicated powders or creams to disguise the resultant skin colour are an asset. These can also be used to hide any temporary marks or scabs which have been caused by the treatment, but which disappear very quickly with proper home-care measures.

During treatment, it is desirable to soothe the skin frequently with lotion to prevent skin reaction, and to cover the area with pads immediately following the application (this can be done on one brow while work is progressing on the second brow). This is very effective in reducing the occurrence of both erythema and oedema (swelling and inflammation). The eye area can react severely to epilation treatment, even if every care is taken, and, therefore, initial treatments should be of short duration and the probes very well spaced until reactions are known. Severe headaches may also occur following the application, and so it is perhaps wiser to suggest that epilation of the brows is contra-indicated for migraine sufferers. Then if, after discussion, the client still wishes to proceed with the treatment, she does so fully aware of the risk involved.

Thus, it can be seen that the work is difficult and a few problems in applying the treatment may be encountered. However, the results are normally excellent and can provide the clients with the permanent solution they are seeking. It is especially rewarding for the really hirsute woman or for the very dark haired individual, whose brows always looked untidy and ungroomed.

TREATMENT OF BREAST HAIRS

Hairs can grow between the breasts as well as on the soft breast tissue itself, but the most common area of growth is around the pigmented skin of the areola and nipple. Hairs here can be extremely strong and difficult to remove, and, therefore, treatment in this area can be somewhat painful, quite apart from being rather embarrassing. So tact, diplomacy and sympathetic handling are needed, in addition to the usual practical skills.

Every effort should be made to put the client at her ease and convince her that her problem is, in fact, not unusual or weird, but rather a commonplace occurrence among women.

If the hair growth is excessive and no evident cause is apparent, then medical advice should be sought, for, as has been seen, many physical conditions can cause a hair growth such as this to occur. The Pill has brought about an increased incidence of breast hair problems among younger women, but this may be remedied by altering the type of Pill prescribed or the form of contraception used. Unfortunately, it is difficult to assess beforehand those women for whom increased levels of oestrogen (the female hormone) will result in the growth of unwanted hair, since the effects are only evident after the body has been exposed to the increased levels for a sustained period. In the same way, hair problems which occur from natural causes may only develop after the second or third pregnancy, in many instances.

The technique involved in treating hairs on the breast in no way differs from treatment in any other soft, fleshy area, except that the hairs are often abnormally strong and deeply placed in the skin. However, they are still structured in the same way as strong hairs elsewhere and are of only a superficial nature in the skin tissues, being in no way involved with the milk ducts of the breast. The client, therefore, can be assured that treatment of these unwanted hairs will not harm her breasts in any way, nor diminish sensitivity of the nipple, nor affect her ability to breast-feed babies. Women present many reasons for not having sought help with their breast hair problem earlier, embarrassment being the main cause, and will often seek the reassurance from the electrologist and an explanation of the cause of the problem. In fact, the incidence of hairs around the nipples is surprisingly common, and this should be made clear to the client to put her mind at rest. As the client has probably had to gather her courage to actually seek help for her problem, she should be handled with understanding and encouragement and in no way be made to feel embarrassed.

Application

First, the client should be asked to remove her bra and slip and change into a clinic robe, to permit the treatment to take place without the need for embarrassing repositioning. She should then be settled in the treatment chair which should be set at a semi-reclining angle. The operator has

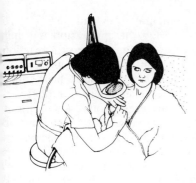

BREAST HAIR—WORKING POSITION

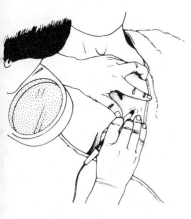

WORK ON BREAST HAIRS

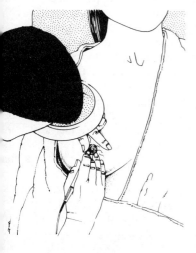

WORK ON NIPPLE HAIRS

to position herself close to the client in order to reach the treatment area, and should probe in the direction of the hair follicles (normally from the opposite side of the client). This enables the client to remain reasonably modestly covered, exposing only that area under immediate attention.

The hairs around the nipples are usually strong and horny in nature and the skin is soft. This calls for the use of a rigid needle such as a .004 Ferrie steel needle. Insulated steel needles may also be used, and these do reduce the initial skin reaction (erythema) quite dramatically, although their increased length makes them less rigid and so a little harder to handle, especially on individuals with a full bust, where the skin is resilient and resists the follicle probe. Operators must work with the needle they feel most at home with, since control over the probe is a most essential factor in breast hair work.

The probe angles may be very varied, particularly if the hairs have previously been plucked repeatedly, causing follicle distortion. Probes may be very upright, steeply angled, or similar to follicle angles on other fleshy areas of the body, that is contoured to the shape of the body. The softness and fleshiness of the breast tissue means that the operator will get very litle guidance as to follicle depth since this is normally provided by the almost imperceptible resistance experienced when the base of the follicle is reached. So, without help from this response, the operator's sense of touch must be excellent and work should be completed very carefully. The first hairs removed should be closely scrutinized to assess follicle depth. In many cases, the stubbornness of the hairs will provide a guide as to the current intensity needed and the angle and depth of the probe required, always bearing in mind the limiting factor of skin sensitivity. For, if these points have not been correctly assessed at the initial inspection then *the hairs will not come out*, but remain very firmly attached. As with basic epilation, the initial probes are used to determine what is needed to produce effective removal without skin damage. Because hairs are in a sensitive skin area, where skin tolerance and the client's capacity for pain impose considerable limitations on the application procedure, they may regrow several times.

Although the client wishes to have this treatment completed, it will not be pleasant and so all possible measures should be taken to minimize discomfort. Treatments should be booked in half-hour sessions, although only a part of this time will be involved with actual treatment application.

Careful pretreatment measures and liberal use of soothing lotions during the application will help to reduce discomfort and minimize skin reaction. There *will* be a reaction to epilation in this area and this must be explained to the client. Small blood spots may form at the mouths of the treated follicles if the hairs are very strong. These minute scabs are part of the healing process; they must not be interfered with, but allowed to disappear naturally. This may take a week or so. Not all clients get this reaction, but it is a wise precaution to warn clients of the possibility, so that they do not become anxious if these temporary marks appear.

If **strong nipple hairs** and **finer breast hair** are present together, the two types of growth can be treated alternately in one treatment session to ease the client's discomfort. This may involve a change in needle diameter as well as adjustment of the current intensity, but it is worthwhile as it extends the client's capacity for treatment. At this stage of her experience, the operator will probably be working with higher current intensities, used for only a fraction of a second (high–fast method). Using this method, adjustments to current intensities will probably be made by varying the length of time the finger button or foot-switch is depressed. Likewise, the operator's increased skill will have considerably reduced the need for different diameter needles and much work will be completed with a .004 Ferrie needle or an insulated steel needle. The latter is usually equivalent to a .004 or .005 Ferrie needle, but is gradually becoming available in a range of diameters.

Applications on hairs growing **around the nipple** should be well spaced in order to avoid converging heat reactions which might result in inflammation, swelling or white ringing. Since the hairs typically grow in very close proximity to each other, appearing as two, or even three hairs from one follicle in some cases, it is sometimes difficult to do this, especially as the client would most likely prefer to have all the hairs cleared from an area at one time. This is where tact and good client handling abilities come to the fore: it should be gently but firmly made plain to the client that the restriction is *absolutely necessary* in order to ensure excellent final results without skin marking. As the client will not thank the operator for any damage or permanent scarring, it is important that the electrologist stand her ground. Naturally both the operator and the client want the fastest possible results, but not at the expense of the operator's professional reputation.

In fact, it may not be advisable to treat **excessive** breast hair in a normal electrology clinic: rather, it should be undertaken under medical supervision in a hospital or private clinic. In any event, the electrologist has the choice of whether to treat or not. If it is thought that more hairs may grow than can be removed because of some physical disturbance, hormonal abnormality, drug medication, or sexual abnormality, the possible success that can be achieved must be explained tactfully to the client. In this way, the client will not expect too much from the treatment, and is less likely to be disappointed with results or disillusioned with the electrologist. In advanced work, honesty about the possible results is essential: clients are usually delighted with results, although there are cases where success is only partial and the operator should be conscious of this point. It often happens, however, that the client is more satisfied with the results than the operator, perhaps because of professional pride.

As breast hair removal can be either a relatively small task or a long-term project, depending on the density and stubbornness of the hairs, the treatment should be offered and charged for on an individual appointment basis of half-hour sessions, rather than as a complete task, as is the case with other advanced work such as removal of hairs from moles. As it is difficult to calculate how many treatments may be required, this is a fairer system for both the client and the operator. If regrowth is not excessive, an early result is achieved and the client does not have to pay for unnecessary work. If, on the other hand, hairs prove very stubborn, the operator covers the extra time required. The work then becomes worthwhile as, compared with normal epilation, it is charged for at perhaps twice the rate per session.

If the client has just a **few breast hairs** which are not too closely spaced and can all be removed in one or two sessions (first one breast, then the other, being treated), only one or two repeat sessions will be needed to clear the regrowth. These appointments can be made as the regrowth hairs emerge, normally six to eight weeks after the initial treatment, although it can be much longer than this, depending on the follicle's recovery rate. If the hairs have grown because of disturbance or hormonal imbalance, however, regrowth may be faster than this.

All these elements are unknown factors when treatment begins, and the operator can only be guided by her experience of previous cases. It is extremely valuable to have observed treatment of breast hairs by an experienced teacher within the training situation, and to have watched a complete treatment programme. When gaining experience in basic techniques, it is well worth persuading an experienced practitioner to permit you to observe her at work to see how the treatment can best be accomplished. Because of the extremely delicate and embarrassing nature of the treatment, permission to observe may be hard to obtain. However, many clients, who are not too modest by nature, will be willing to co-operate, if the point is made that it is the only way the trainee can learn how to perform this difficult work, and so to be able to help other women with breast hair problems. If observation does not prove possible, then a fellow student with this condition may be found who will offer herself as a guinea-pig to provide the necessary first experience, so vital before starting work on a paying client. Electrologists who train in a clinic under a tutor will certainly be able to observe advanced techniques being applied first hand as part of the normal clinic practice. Likewise, in a technical college, clients with a range of hair problems will be obtained to act as models to extend the students' experience. If the training situation does not provide the opportunity to observe work of this type, however, the trainee must make the effort to find a means of gaining this experience before embarking on professional practice. Experienced operators in the professional associations will often be willing to pass on their expertise to the younger members. Working alongside a highly qualified and experienced electrologist is the best way of learning these skills, and is of inestimable value to the newly qualified operator who hopes to be able to offer these treatments in the future. If a busy operator can be persuaded to help, it must be expected that her time and effort should be paid for. The knowledge acquired has a real commercial value, increasing, as it does, the earning capacity of the operator, and, therefore, an investment in time and money to gain the skills needed is both necessary and worthwhile.

TREATMENT OF THREAD VEINS (DILATED CAPILLARIES), SPIDER NAEVI AND BLOOD SPOTS

Once again, the real skill involved here does not lie in the actual technique, but in both knowing where to apply the current and how much current to use to effect a decrease in the capillary structure without unduly harming the skin, and also in recognizing when treatment would be not only pointless or even harmful to the client, but, perhaps, likely to provide only a temporary answer because of the weakness of the tissues themselves.

Causes of Capillary Damage

FRAGILE SKIN

Capillary damage resulting in thread veins, dilated capillaries, blood spots, or small spider naevi are most often a sign of fragile skin. Such skin is unable to withstand exposure to harsh elements such as extremes of weather, rough daily treatment, or the use of strong or caustic cosmetic or washing routines. *This skin weakness cannot be cured by minor cosmetic electrology used to seal off the offending capillaries visible on the skin's surface.* The capillaries are there as a sign of the weakness, and, because of this weakness, they will constantly re-form, not because of any fault in the application, but as a result of the inherent problem from which the client suffers—skin fragility and thin structure. If the capillary weakness is extensive, with no defined boundaries, then treatment could do more harm than good. Since nothing can cure the weakness, the results are bound to be poor, and overall appearance at the conclusion of the treatment could be worse than at the start.

INJURY

Individuals with thicker, tougher skin seldom suffer from capillary damage, and, if they do, it is usually as a direct result of an injury to the area causing capillary dilation and rupture. Since these ruptured vessels are not due to an overall weakness, treatment of them is successful and the results normally permanent.

RECURRING PROBLEM

If capillary damage arises from a steadily recurring problem—for instance, a spider naevus caused by careless plucking of the eyebrows (picking up skin in addition to the elected hair)—then the cause of the problem must be eliminated if at all possible to prevent the condition recurring. In the same way, blood spots found on pressure areas, such as the bridge of the nose where glasses rest, will normally recur in time, because the skin has been previously damaged and cannot be repaired by short wave diathermy treatment. Only the offending spot of stagnant, trapped blood that had ruptured into the tissues can be permanently removed.

Blood spots and thread-like veins can occur on any area of the face excessively exposed to sun or wind. The tip of the nose is an especially common site for blood spots, being prone to sunburn, windburn and peeling, and this is one of the worst areas in which to achieve success because of its continual exposure to these harsh elements. The blood spot or veins formed here are normally due to a breakdown in the skin's integrity and strength as a result of injury or damage (for example, blistering and peeling caused by bad sunburn). These conditions can also occur around the nostril area, brought about by blowing the nose hard when suffering from colds or allergies (for example, hay fever), which places the tiny blood vessels of the nostrils under stress.

HIGH BLOOD PRESSURE

If the skin is generally very vascular, florid in colour, with bulbous blood vessels protruding from the surface, then the problem may be due to high blood pressure. A prime cause of the high colour seen on mature women is high blood pressure, sometimes associated with being overweight. In this instance although the unsightly veins could be treated, the underlying problem cannot be resolved by the electrologist; the skin is only responding naturally to the stimuli received via the bloodstream—hormone messengers prescribe the degree of blood vessel dilation (expansion) needed to accommodate the volume and rate of flow of blood in the surface and subcutaneous blood vessels. Medical attention must be sought.

So, total success in the treatment of 'red veins' (as they are often simply described to the client), cannot be assured and for this reason many electrologists prefer not to treat the condition at all. However, where the problem would seem to be the result of an injury or carelessness, good results can be obtained. The electrologist's skill lies in deciding which conditions will benefit from treatment and which will not, and then proceeding with the treatment, all the time watching the skin's reaction to avoid further damage.

It must be reiterated that short wave diathermy current is itself a destructive force, able, through its cauterizing effects, to render hair follicles incapable of producing new hairs, and now this destructive action is to be used to eliminate ruptured blood vessels without further damage being caused. Naturally, this is not possible. The whole art of capillary treatment is, in fact, the ability to maximize the effect of this heat sealing and coagulating current without causing skin tissue damage.

There can be no guarantee of complete success in the treatment of capillaries, and this must be understood by the client at the outset so that her expectations are not too high and the electrologist's professional reputation is protected. Even so, most clients are delighted with the final results and feel that the effort, time and expense involved have been worthwhile.

Thread Veins (Dilated Capillaries)—Application

When dealing with fragile skin, the first step in mapping out treatment is to consider what has happened to the small surface capillaries. Normally positioned in the *dermal* layers of the skin, the small capillaries dilate (expand) and rupture into the *surface* skin layers, seeping through them in a thread-like formation easily visible through the epidermal layers. This blood cannot flow away back into the skin's general vascular system: it becomes trapped and stagnant, and turns a bluish colour. As well as this trapped blood, dilated blood vessels are also visible, appearing like a tracery of interconnected veins and capillaries, sometimes with patches of congested vessels, which look like blood spots in the densest areas. The overall appearance, then, is one of high colour with the varicosed, bulbous areas standing out to add further to the imperfection.

Within this area of dilated blood vessels, individual vessels can be cauterized—that is, the trapped blood in between the layers of skin can be treated with tiny amounts of short wave diathermy current. A minute bruise forms, which then disperses and is reabsorbed into the body in the same way as a natural bruise. As the skin is open during this process, there is a constant risk of skin infection, and, therefore, stringent hygiene measures must be enforced during and after treatment.

The tiny vessels are 'tapped' along their visible length, working inwards from their outermost point or end towards the larger or more livid and important blood vessels: it may well be that these cannot be treated as they are part of the actual vascular supply. A fine steel needle and a minute amount of current (far less than is used in hair destruction) is used to lightly seal the blood vessel and cauterize the surface. The needle point can be directed into the small vessel without causing pain, and this keeps the diathermy current below the surface, thus minimizing the skin reaction while effectively coagulating the blood in the vessel. On application, or discharge of the current, the skin immediately blanches and the blood seems to disappear ahead along the tiny vessel. This is a straightforward heat or burn reaction, with the current being carried forward by the blood fluid in the capillary but it is most important that great vigilance be paid when applying the current, and the intensity adjusted whenever necessary.

Careless work can result in white depigmented areas (white shiny patches) leaving a disfigurement worse than the original capillary dilation. These burn scars are similar to those resulting from excessive use of current and 'white ringing' in electrology, only worse, as the current has been intentionally applied to the skin itself. The hard, horny, keratinized surface of the skin reacts strongly to diathermy application, resulting in instant blistering if the current intensity is too high. Since the surface of the skin has little natural moisture, to avoid this problem the needle point has only to be slipped under the skin a fraction to reach the moisture of the blood fluid to which the current is attracted.

A fine, but rigid steel needle of medium diameter, which is not unduly flexible, is used to accomplish the tapping. It may be an ordinary Ferrie needle of .004 to .005 diameter or a more rigid, longer needle, again of steel but with a very sharp point. This enables the needle to enter the capillary easily and to slide into it a little way so as to reach and seal the vessel without burning the skin. The current is applied fractionally, in tiny amounts, along the length of the capillary (hence the description, 'tapping') to complete the cautery. The skin overlying the blood vessel appears completely transparent, but will often be hard to pierce, so a sharp point on the needle is essential. Ferrie needles have sharp points, but they become slightly dulled by usage, and, therefore, only new needles should be used, and these must be meticulously sterilized prior to use to prevent infection; or, if available, the disposable sterile needles *Sterex* should be used. These are the ideal choice for the job.

The vessels undergoing treatment should be well spaced, and as soon as the skin appears irritated or very red, then treatment should stop, the skin covered with damp pads soaked in soothing lotion and another area treated. Until the

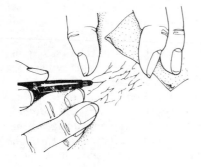

TAPPING ALONG A
DILATED CAPILLARY

skin's healing capacity is known, periods of treatment should be short and the applications well spaced on the most superficial vessels in the less prominent areas. The skin heals with a series of very small scabs, like scratches: *these must be permitted to drop off naturally, and not encouraged off by the client.* This should be stressed to the clients along with the need to treat their skin gently while the course of treatment is in progress. This will be good training for clients in learning to treat their fragile skins a little more kindly, thereby helping to prevent recurrence of the problem in the future.

If treatment has consisted of coagulating a whole area of tiny capillaries, these will heal in the form of running scratches which soon disappear as the scabs dry and drop off. This process can be aided by applying drying and healing *powder* immediately after the application to camouflage the skin, protect it from transient (airborne) bacteria and start the healing process. The area should not be cleansed or washed for at least twenty-four hours, nor interfered with or covered with make-up until the tiny scabs form. The erythema will soon disperse, and, although the area may be hot and irritated for a few hours, by the next day it should be calm, with the forming scabs as the only sign of treatment. Medicated make-up can then be used following the drying powder application to hide the scratches, but it must be cleansed off gently and thoroughly to avoid disrupting the healing process. Removing scabs prematurely may result in infection which can lead to dehydration and pitting of the skin.

One of the main problems is the maintenance of skin hygiene when the client leaves the clinic, and the co-operation of the client here is vital. The home-care measures should be carefully explained, and written down on a salon card to serve as a guide and a reminder. The necessary products—soothing lotions, drying and healing powders, medicated creams (if infection does occur), etc.—should be provided by the clinic or advice given as to where they may be purchased. Preferably, they should be sold by the clinic, simply to ensure that they are available for the client's use and there is no possible excuse for not following the prescribed skin hygiene routine at home. The daily application of drying powder to speed the scabbing process and hasten desiccation and desquamation (skin drying and scaling off) is essential to success.

If only a **few dilated capillaries** or thread veins needed treatment initially, a reassessment can be

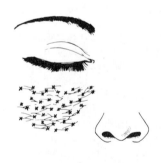

CAPILLARY TREATMENT
STAGE 1

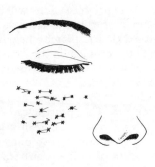

CAPILLARY TREATMENT
STAGE 2

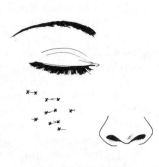

CAPILLARY TREATMENT
STAGE 3

made two or three weeks after the first application to determine what further treatment is needed. It may be that three weeks are sufficient to allow the skin to accept further treatment, or a much longer healing gap may be required. The longer the skin can be given to recover, the better will be the overall result. By seeing the client after two or three weeks, the electrologist will be able to make an assessment of the progress so far, reassure the client and at the same time make a forward appointment to deal with the remaining capillaries. Even a small area of dilated capillaries benefits from being treated in two stages rather than in one application, as this appears to overstress the skin's capacity for recovery.

Once the skin has healed, the remaining capillaries can be treated, but the electrologist should at all times be mindful that the skin, as well as being inherently fragile, is still recovering from the trauma of the short wave diathermy application. If, for any reason, she considers the repeat application to be premature, she should postpone the treatment until the skin is in a more healthy condition. A really severe erythema reaction, blistering, discomfort or soreness would be the signs to look for here.

Periodic checking on the condition of the skin and the way the disappearance of the capillaries is progressing is useful to the operator and welcomed by the client. The checking takes only a minute and yet it is important because it provides an opportunity to see that the skin has not become infected, thereby requiring a change from protective to antiseptic and antibacterial measures. If the client cannot attend the clinic for any reason, she should be asked to indicate her progress by telephone. This precaution not only safeguards the client's skin but also the electrologist's professional reputation.

The skin is extremely adept at healing itself, quickly forming scabs and sealing off the area, while it heals internally. However, if bacteria do enter the area, an infection can result and must be dealt with. Some clients are much more susceptible to sepsis than others, and this should be ascertained prior to treatment, so that additional medicated measures can be taken, if indeed treatment is undertaken at all. Electrologists do not work in sterile surroundings such as are found in hospitals, even though they work with rigid attention to maintaining a state of asepsis. So the risk of airborne bacteria is always present, especially with a regular flow of clients coming into the clinic from the outside world. The greatest risk, as we have seen, comes when the client leaves the clinic and returns to her home or work environment. However, once the tiny scabs have formed, the worst danger is over and, unless they are scratched off, the skin is protected from that stage onwards and heals very rapidly. If a scab is removed, leaving an open area, the aftercare measures outlined above can be reintroduced, using drying, medicated powder until a new scab is formed.

As capillary conditions can vary so tremendously, both in terms of their severity and their rate of healing, it is preferable to charge for vein treatment per appointment or treatment session. Again, this is specialized work and should be costed at a much higher rate than basic electrology—the charge is normally twice the basic rate for epilation. It is often sensible to wait until after the initial consultation before advising clients of the cost of their treatment, so that a reasonably accurate estimate of the amount of money and time needed to resolve the problem can be given. The number of appointments necessary to complete the treatment should be made quite plain, and the overall time-span discussed.

If **capillary damage is extensive**, involving many parts of the face, nose and lower cheeks, then weekly or fortnightly appointments can be given and each area can be treated in rotation at a separate appointment. By careful attendance to clinic records and obvious visible signs from the skin, both *new areas* and those ready for *re-treatment* may be dealt with simultaneously as the appointments progress. With experience, the electrologist will be able to tell exactly when a capillary area is ready for further treatment: the skin will appear healthy and be a good colour, the tissues will be firm and elastic and the normal blood supply minus the dilated capillary will have returned to the area. All that will then remain are fragmented sections of the previously continuous, intact blood vessel, and these tiny areas of blood can be treated individually in the same way, but using even less current intensity than on the initial application. If re-treatment is carried out on a capillary prematurely then the fragmented sections will not have re-formed, and a false impression of progress will be created. These blood dots *will* reappear eventually, and it is better if they are treated at the correct time, rather than treating them too soon and causing them to appear at a later stage, since this will only annoy the client and make the treatment seem ineffective.

As work should progress systematically, with areas of skin gradually clearing and recovering, from the outermost points of the condition in towards the worst affected areas, these will gradually seem to become more prominent. This is simply because the most bulbous, bulging capillaries then stand out and are very apparent when not set against the general high colour of surrounding vascularity. Clients may feel that the problem is becoming worse and not better, and must be encouraged to be patient and see the entire programme through to the end before they judge results. However, it sometimes happens that clients are really only worried about one or two very visible capillaries in prominent places, such as under the eye, and, when these have been removed, they are satisfied and do not wish to continue with further applications. The operator should not press the client; if the operator offers her professional skill only when it is sought, then the client is more likely to return at any future date when she needs help. Just as it is the client's skin and imperfection, so it is also her choice to decide when to continue with treatment and when to stop.

Spider Naevi—Application

The spider naevus has a central blood spot with tiny capillaries radiating from it resembling a spider's legs. These are dealt with in a similar manner to thread veins with very good results—normally total disappearance. If the spider naevus is caused by an injury, such as a blow to the area or catching the skin with tweezers, or follows the removal of a cyst or a deep-seated skin infection (a boil or abscess), then the result of treatment will be permanent and the naevus should not re-form. However, if the spider naevus is present as a result of general skin weakness, increased blood pressure, overall vascularity of the skin, etc., then, although the treated spider naevus may not reform, further naevi may break out close by.

Spider naevi can be found anywhere on the face or body, and are often seen in conjunction with areas of dilated capillaries, high colour, and so on. They can be treated in association with thread veins if this is the case, being themselves only a series of capillaries which converge to form a blood spot or area of trapped blood.

Multiple spider naevi often occur during pregnancy as a direct result of increased blood pressure and volume experienced at this time. The naevi will be tiny, not usually defined, and assume a star-like form of running red threads or dots. They can be present on the hands, face and, in some cases, on the body as well. *These small spider naevi should not be treated as they normally disappear spontaneously a short while after the birth.* If this regression (reduction in size or disappearance) does not occur, and they seem to have become a permanent skin imperfection despite the return to normal blood pressure levels, then they may be treated by the electrologist a few months after the birth.

Both dilated capillaries and naevi may also be evident on the legs as a result of strain and inefficient blood circulation. Individuals who spend a lot of time standing at work, especially if they are confined to one area rather than moving about (such as serving behind a counter), seem to be particularly prone to circulatory problems. They suffer both internally with varicose veins, and superficially with thread veins, spider naevi, etc. When the veins carrying blood back to the heart become congested because of a weakness in the valves of the major leg veins, then these veins swell, ache and may protrude. Varicose veins can be seen deeply situated in the leg, clearly evident because of the dark-blue colour of the stagnant, deoxygenated blood they carry. In severe cases, they are also visible as dark-bluish veins which protrude on to the surface of the skin, presenting a bulbous, swollen appearance. *If spider naevi or thread veins are present among the varicose veins, they must not be treated, as to do so could be very dangerous for the client.* The varicosity indicates the circulatory defect, and the surface rupture is simply another aspect of the problem, yet intrinsically linked to it.

When dilated capillaries are sealed off, the blood supply in the area is diminished, and the blood supplying the skin tissues in the area has to find another route. It is to be hoped that this route lies through established blood vessels positioned *deeper* in the skin, so that other superficial blood vessels are not overstressed by the additional load, and themselves subsequently dilate or rupture. If the skin is frail, thin and suffers from poor circulation already, or if the underlying vessels are overstressed and inefficient (as with varicose veins), then there is no point in treating the capillary rupture. In fact, treatment has occasionally been found to make the condition far worse, causing areas not previously affected by the vascularity to become traced with dilated capillaries, blood spots and naevi.

Electrologists must, therefore, know when to advise the client against capillary treatment. If they feel, for example, that treatment of a surface imperfection could aggravate or worsen a serious condition of varicose veins, with the possible risk of a thrombosis (blood clot), they must advise against treatment. Interfering with the body's essential blood circulation not only runs the risk of inducing an embolism, where a moving blood clot could lodge in any organ of the body, but could also cause ulcers to form in the area of treatment. As the skin's circulation is already impaired, its capacity to heal is very poor, and infection resulting from capillary treatment could lead to skin ulceration and sores that will not heal. These may already be present if the individual suffers from varicose veins, but, in any event, would be worsened by diathermy applications used to seal off and remove ruptured surface vessels.

Treatment of spider naevi is more or less the same no matter where in the body they are found, and one application is normally sufficient to remove them. If there are several positioned close together, then the applications should be well spaced, some of the capillaries being treated at one appointment and the rest at the following appointment, at least six weeks later. It is wise to draw up a treatment plan only after an initial inspection of the condition, and not to commit oneself to treatment guarantees over the telephone, as imperfections of this type often turn out to be more complicated than clients realize.

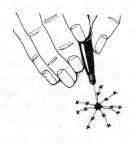

TREATMENT OF
SPIDER NAEVUS 'LEGS'

The 'legs' (or radiating capillaries) of the 'spider' (or central blood spot) are treated by working from the outside in towards the central concentration of blood. Using the same technique as for thread veins, the blood vessels are lightly touched, tapped and blanched along their length; the colour disappears on contact with the heat of the diathermy current. The intensity used is very low, sufficient only to cauterize the vessel, not to burn the skin. When all the capillaries have been treated, the area will appear blanched, white, raised and a little swollen, with the remaining blood spot at the centre. With a small naevus, the current running ahead along the small vessels, carried by the blood, will often make the central spot disappear spontaneously, coagulated by the converging applications of current from the legs of the naevus, and it may be that no further treatment will be required. The electrologist will be able to tell from experience whether the central spot is likely to re-form after the skin has re-

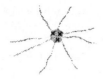

TREATMENT OF
SPIDER NAEVUS 'BODY'

covered and whether it should be treated independently. The swelling and blanching of the skin, in fact, hide the nature and density of the spot and present a false picture. In most cases, it is wiser to err on the side of caution by discharging a tiny amount of current directly into the centre of the remaining blood spot, whereupon it will immediately turn white and the blood colour disappear. The art of successful capillary work is to use the minimum amount of current in exactly the right place, balancing cautery against unnecessary skin damage.

At the follow-up appointment, six weeks after the application, any remaining signs of the capillary weakness will show up, and these can then be treated. If a single spider naevus or blood spot is treated, then a charge for the complete task is the normal procedure, and this charge usually covers any follow-up work. Although the actual treatment may take only a few minutes, it is normally offered as a half-hour appointment, and charged at the minor cosmetic electrology rate. This allows the operator to complete the work without pressure from subsequent appointments, and allows time to settle the client, explain procedures, provide short pauses during treatment, if necessary, and explain home-care measures in detail.

Again, home-care hygiene must match clinic care if infection, poor healing and scarring are not to result. The client should be advised to dry the area with medicated powder to help scab formation and, through desiccation, to speed healing and prohibit the growth of bacteria. In a concentrated area such as a spider naevus, the skin takes a lot of punishment from the diathermy application and must be helped to heal. Care must be taken not to subject the skin to strain by harsh, vigorous washing and cleansing. Soothing lotion and drying medicated powder should be used during the first twenty-four hours to protect the skin, and after that normal cleansing procedures may be followed. If infection does set in, germicidal measures of a drying nature can be adopted; creams should be avoided if possible as these delay the scabbing process. If clients are made aware of the importance of their home-care measures in achieving overall success, they are seldom careless over this point, having their own best interests at heart.

Blood Spots—Application

Blood spots are concentrations of blood, present on the surface of the skin, overlaid with a translucent skin layer through which the blood shows vividly, and are usually bright red in colour, like the centre of a naevus. They should only be treated if they are small and superficial in nature, but if they appear like a protrusion of a deeper blood vessel pushing through to the surface of the skin, *they must on no account be treated*. If any doubt exists as to the nature of the blood spot, medical advice must be sought prior to treatment.

Treatment of blood spots is very similar to that of spider naevi. However, as there are no 'legs' to treat first, hence no converging current to start off the coagulation of the central blood accumulation, the central area must withstand quite a large concentration of current in one small place. It could, therefore, easily suffer skin damage and become depigmented, forming a white patch on healing. So, larger blood spots should be treated in two or even three sessions, in order that the skin damage can be monitored by the electrologist and the applications adjusted accordingly.

Small blood spots can be treated by touching the outer rim (or perimeter) all around with tiny amounts of short wave diathermy current. The current flows inwards, attracted by the moistness of the blood fluid, the colour disappears and the area becomes white and raised. The central area can then be coagulated if necessary, and the whole area soothed and covered with pads to reduce immediate swelling and colour. The skin responds quickly to the trauma of the application and a fierce colour or erythema reaction forms around the treated area, which can be camouflaged by flesh-tinted, medicated powder. Home-care is identical to that described for the spider naevus.

Larger blood spots can first be reduced in size by treating their boundaries, again working inwards, directing the needle angle in towards just below the centre of the spot. If the blood spot is thought of as a diamond, the angle of the needle would be pointing towards the base point of the diamond. This concentrates the current towards the core of the blood spot, and contains its damaging effects away from the dry skin tissue. The remaining surface area of the spot can then be treated in a dotted fashion, leaving some areas untreated. The entire blood spot will seem to disappear, but will, in fact, re-emerge in a patchy fashion in the weeks following treatment. This remaining fragmented blood can then be treated six weeks or more after the first application, to complete the task. The reasons for splitting the treatment up in this way—less discomfort, less

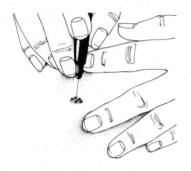

LARGER BLOOD SPOT TREATMENT
STAGE 1

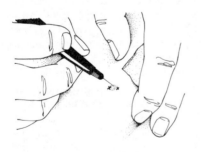

LARGER BLOOD SPOT TREATMENT
STAGE 2

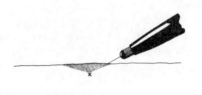

DIAMOND SHAPE
FOR NEEDLE ANGLE

risk of colour loss (depigmentation), scar formation or pitting and a decrease in the overall chances of the blood spot re-forming—should all be explained to the client.

TREATMENT OF MOLE HAIRS

Unsightly hairs protruding from moles cause considerable distress, but can be helped by the electrologist if she first receives medical approval to treat the condition. The electrologist is in a difficult position as far as treating mole hairs without medical approval is concerned, however, because she is not legally covered by insurance on the very rare occasion of a mole proving to be cancerous and interference with it being considered a contributory factor.

As has been stated, moles are benign tumours (see Chapter 6), that is they are normally inactive, but are implicated as secondary cancers in rare instances where the individual already has a primary cancer in another part of the body. However, the electrologist is not in a position to know whether a mole is benign or not, or has any potential for becoming cancerous if interfered with. Only medical investigation can furnish this knowledge. Electrologists must always err on the side of caution whenever there is a risk, however slight.

Application

When medical approval is given, however, treatment may be undertaken. Since most of a mole's colour is associated with the roots of the hairs growing from it, the colour will decrease in intensity once the hairs are removed. Thus, the mole will become far less apparent simply by removing the hairs. If the client wishes to be free of both the mole and the hairs, she should be advised to have it excised surgically, performed under a local anaesthetic in medical surroundings; it is a painless procedure.

The hairs are deeply placed within the core of the mole and converge towards the centre, making the probing angles almost upright on occasions. This convergence means that the skin will be subjected to a considerable accumulation of current as each hair root is treated. Although the hair follicles on the surface of the mole may appear well spaced, their strong roots are not, and the underlying tissues could suffer damage if subjected to too much current. So, hairs chosen for the initial removal should be spaced out, leaving the remaining hairs for a subsequent treatment,

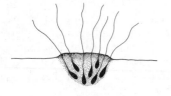

MOLE HAIRS:
CONVERGING ROOTS

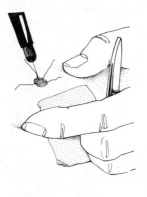

ACTUAL TREATMENT
OF MOLE HAIRS

after two to three weeks have elapsed. Naturally, if only three or four hairs in total are present, then these can be removed in one application, and their regrowth treated when it appears, normally six to eight weeks later. The number of hairs growing from a mole is deceptive. Often the client will say that she has only a few hairs to be removed, but, on close inspection, it turns out to be many more, although the prominent, strong ones of which the client is aware may well be only a few in number.

If a number of hairs are present and need to be dealt with in several sessions, the most apparent ones' should be dealt with first. Naturally, the electrologist must wait until the client has become adjusted to the epilation treatment before starting work on the strongest and most painful hairs. Hairs in moles often grow quite out of character to the client's normal hair, and can be multiple hairs (multi-germini—two or three hairs growing from one follicle), or be distorted and excessively strong. The hair sheaths can become dense structures, closely surrounding the hair root and completely filling the follicle, making probing very difficult. The skin tissues of the mole itself are also different from normal skin, and can be either soft and fleshy or hard and horny in nature. The skin area has to be handled firmly and probing accomplished with a rigid, medium diameter needle, which ideally should be longer than the standard, Ferrie-type needle. A .005 diameter Ferrie needle can be used, but a longer, thinner needle gives the operator more control. Some operators will work with a selection of needles, some of which fit into the Ferrie needle holder chuck, while others fit the smaller aperture of the insulated steel needle holder. The fitting, however, must be very firm and the connection perfect. The variable fitting on some needle holders, which enables them to take a wide range of different diameter needles, is excellent for this type of work, as the spiral connection grasps the needle very firmly and does not allow any unwanted movement to occur. Needles designed for the treatment of moles and mole hairs must be strong in order to take the level of current intensity needed to accomplish destruction of these strong hairs without fracturing. In addition, the needle must be relatively inflexible, otherwise probing becomes very difficult and accuracy in reaching the hair root almost impossible to achieve.

There is very little 'feed back' or feeling of resistance from the base of the follicles of mole hairs, and follicle depth and angle have to be

largely determined by examining the hairs themselves—their size, position, horniness, etc. Initial
examination of the first successfully epilated hair,
and assessment of its condition, acts as a guide for
further applications. Current strength should initially be kept reasonably low until a more accurate assessment of the correct level can be made.
Hairs which have been probed and treated should
be tested for destruction by a gentle, lifting
pressure to see if they come free. *They must not be
tugged out.* If they do not immediately come free
and if the skin appears reasonably calm, they can
be re-treated with a slightly higher current intensity or a fractional prolonging of the time the
current is applied. Then, the intensity and duration of the current application can be adjusted for
work on other hairs on the basis of this knowledge.

Most hairy moles will need several treatments:
the first to clear all the hairs, and subsequent
treatments to deal with the regrowth which is
inevitable due to the strength and nature of the
follicles. Even if only a few hairs are present on a
mole, these will often be grouped in clumps,
making total removal of all the hairs impossible
without causing converging skin reactions. So it is
vital to a successful result that all the hairs are not
treated in one session, in order not to over-tax the
skin.

The usual aftercare measures of applying
drying, healing, medicated powder, both immediately following treatment and at home, to hasten
healing and prevent infection, are necessary. If the
skin of the mole and its surrounding tissue become
sore and slow to heal and dry, then normal
germicidal measures can be used, but this is
seldom necessary.

TREATMENT OF FIBROMA SIMPLEX, PAPILLOMAS AND WARTS

All fibrous growths, whether flat (sessile) or
raised from the surface of the skin (pedunculated—raised on a stalk) are caused by a skin
irregularity often associated with the keratinization process. These fibrous imperfections
become more common with age, so it would
appear that their formation is connected with a
slowing down of the basal rate of mitotic activity
in the skin. As the replacement or growth rate of
the skin slows down, so the incidence of these
imperfections increases. Most of these fibrous

accumulations are simply unsightly or feel unpleasant, but do not appear to be connected to any decrease in skin function. Many of the simple fibrous growths (or **fibroma simplex**) are different in colour and texture from normal skin, and it is this rather than any increase in size or protrusion that makes them apparent. They may become shiny and glassy in appearance and lose colour, appearing as white, raised patches which can be felt as hard, movable lumps or papules in the skin's surface layers, or the skin may become hyperpigmented, assuming a dark red-brown or a dusky, wine colour, often on a naturally florid or ruddy complexion. The skin may retain its normal colour, with the fibroma clearly defined, having a raised border or even attached to the skin by a stalk-like tube of skin. These raised fibroma are more commonly referred to as **pedunculated papillomas**, and may be tiny or grow to a considerable size, with the body of the growth being the size of a pea. These imperfections can often be seen on the faces of elderly people, and can be a nuisance if they are close to the eyes or mouth, quite apart from being unattractive in themselves.

If the fibrous growths take a multiple form, such as is commonly seen on the neck, they are known as **skin tags** and can develop what is known as a 'tear drop' formation, denoting their shape and position. These skin tags are a very common factor associated with skin ageing, and only really cause distress if they are hyperpigmented and, therefore, more obvious. The fact that they are so much associated with ageing is a major reason why mature clients dislike their presence and are anxious to have them removed. Skin tags are like tiny flaps of skin, shaped like a tear or diamond, which are attached to the main surface of the skin by a narrow area of skin tissue. Like all fibrous growths, they receive their blood supply and nourishment from the dermal layers of the skin; indeed they are like a protrusion of the dermis, pushed through the epidermal layer.

The actual principle by which these tiny, unwanted growths are removed is to cut off their blood supply, whereupon they wither, atrophy, dry up and drop off. This is accomplished by accurately cauterizing the area of skin by which they are attached to the main surface of the skin, i.e. applying short wave diathermy current to their stalk or skin attachment. Naturally, fibrous growths, papillomas and skin tags are much easier to treat if they are pedunculated, because then the growth itself need not be treated, only its attachment which is normally the smallest area of the growth, and the client does not experience any severe discomfort.

If fibromas are large and present a well-defined area of hard, keratinized skin tissue, they may well have a good vascular and nervous supply, which would make them too painful for removal in this way. These should be treated medically, excised (surgically cut away) under a local anaesthetic in a sterile hospital situation. Stitches may, in fact, also be needed. (Any moles (pigmented fibromas), hairy moles or warts which are of size to cause severe discomfort if treated by minor cosmetic electrology methods should also be dealt with in the hospital situation.)

Most of the tiny skin growths the electrologist is asked to treat are of a much more minor nature and are more like tiny projections of the epidermis. For this reason they are sometimes known as **epidermal cysts** and can in fact be cysts, that is, skin debris or sebum trapped in a blind duct in the skin, which the surface skin layers overlay until a lump is formed. There are many variations of these fibrous imperfections and they are described in many ways, all of them correct and interchangeable in medical terms. The name by which a condition is known and described relates to its cause, its form and structure, and its history if this is clear cut.

Warts are skin overgrowths as well, but, although very similar in appearance and form to other fibromas, they are caused by a virus infection and are infectious or contagious. They are capable of vanishing spontaneously, and many unusual methods (home remedies or power of the mind) are used to try to accomplish this. Electrologists should advise clients to seek medical treatment for persistent warts and only then, if all other methods of hastening their departure fail, should epilation treatment be undertaken. Great care must be taken with sterilization routines to prevent cross-infection. The operator should avoid direct contact with the warts by the use of tissues and pads, in order to diminish the risk of being infected personally. Multiple wart formations seldom require a lot of treatment if the individual pin-like heads are treated progressively, as the instance of spontaneous disappearance after the first few applications is remarkable. Treatment of warts is identical to that of fibromas, though the skin is normally hornier and requires a stronger current for successful removal. Fortunately, treatment of warts does not cause much discomfort to the client, because, being more keratinized than fleshy, they do not have a well-established vascular and nervous supply.

All abnormalities and deviations from normal skin which the electrologist undertaking minor cosmetic electrology sees at first hand, confirms the fact that the skin is a very complex structure, closely affected by physical health, hormone levels, stress and so on. The link between pigmentation and hormonal activity is clearly seen during pregnancy or any illness connected with a malfunction of an endocrine organ. What is less obvious is the skin's response to ageing, nutritional deficiencies, depression, and anxiety. The operator who progresses into this very complex area of work will become acutely aware of the link between skin imperfections and the health of the individual, and must know when an abnormality would benefit from medical attention. Any excessive skin growth, or change in colour, texture or elasticity comes into this category, and, just as excessive hair growth needs to be looked at carefully, so does an unexpected incidence of fibrous growths, skin tags, pigmented moles or warts.

Again, deciding when to treat, or when a condition warrants medical advice is the most important and difficult part of treating fibrous growths. It is unwise to treat any condition which has the slightest element of risk attached to it, or where results might be unsatisfactory. Only personal experience will build up the knowledge and ability to make these decisions with confidence, and so in the early days caution is essential.

Fibroma Simplex— Application

The simple fibroma, or fibrous growth, is a small mass of horny keratinized tissue, which may or may not have a visible vascular supply. Many small growths have an irregular surface and are raised prominently above the surrounding skin. Fibromas of this type, if small in diameter, respond to short wave diathermy application very well. However, if the fibroma is flat (sessile) but hyperpigmented, therefore visible but not protruding, cosmetic electrology treatment is not ideal as there is little that can be removed or cauterized. The fibrous growth may well grow inwards rather than outwards, and therefore treatment lies outside the scope of the electrologist. Cosmetic electrology works on the principle of removing only that which is unwanted or unnecessary, and in this instance that is not the case.

The raised fibroma or fibrous lump is treated in a similar manner to a blood spot, working inwards from its boundaries, discharging the current into the mass of the tiny growth, just under the surface. A finely pointed needle should be used to combine strength and rigidity, although the needle diameter is unimportant as no follicle probing is being undertaken. The tip of the needle carrying the current should not be placed too deeply into the fibroma, otherwise an indentation or pit in the skin could occur. Treatment should be progressive, so that the surface area of the growth is reduced gradually, by the application of controlled, minute amounts of current, until the skin surface is flat.

The first treatment should cover the entire area of the fibroma, working all around the boundaries, leaving spaces between each application to avoid over-treatment and angling the needle inwards towards just below the centre of the growth. This will reduce the skin tissue from both above and below. The area should be soothed with cooling lotion during and after the treatment, and then covered with a liberal amount of medicated powder. This speeds up the desiccation or skin drying process, and helps the skin tissue to scab and peel off. *This scab must be left to heal and drop off naturally*. This last point is vital to the success of the treatment. When, after four to six weeks, the scab has fallen of naturally, any remaining work can be completed. In this way, the skin will recover properly and over-treatment will be avoided. The skin must be kept dry and covered until the scab forms, and, if the scab is knocked off accidentally, then drying, medicated measures must be reintroduced. The importance of this point must be emphasized to the client. The charge for treatment of these small, raised fibromas usually covers the complete treatment, including the consultation and follow-up appointment.

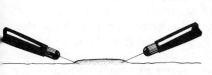

FIBROMA: PROBING ANGLE

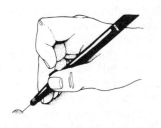

TREATMENT OF INDIVIDUAL
FIBROMA

Pedunculated Papillomas and Skin Tags (Raised Fibrous Growths)—Application

PEDUNCULATED PAPILLOMA

Pedunculated papillomas (growths attached by a stalk to the surface of the skin) are treated by cauterizing their attachment points with small amounts of diathermy current. The operator holds the growth or tag firmly between the fingers, so

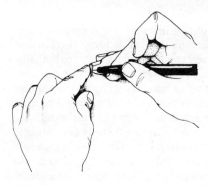

TREATMENT THROUGH THE STALK

MULTIPLE SKIN TAGS

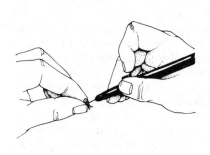

TREATMENT THROUGH THE STALK

that the treatment point is static, and directs the point of a fine needle carefully into the stalk. One or two points of application are usually sufficient to ensure complete cessation of the blood supply. The cautery is then complete, and nature finishes off the task in the next few days or weeks, causing the skin flap or lump to dry up, wrinkle, become like a dry leaf and eventually drop off. Often there is nothing further left to be treated, but this must be checked at a follow-up appointment: it is always better to undertreat, and have to finish off the task later, than over-treat and cause skin damage, pitting, scarring and marking. It is most gratifying to have a client who, at the completion of her treatment, shows absolutely no sign of the work which has been undertaken, and looks as if the imperfection has never existed.

Multiple skin tags, which can be very numerous on some older women, should be treated in several sessions, dealing first with the individual tags which annoy the client most or of which she is most conscious. Although skin tags are fiddling to grasp, the operator must not be afraid of holding them firmly while cauterization takes place. A strong, fine needle is used and only one point of application to the *skin attachment* is needed to accomplish the treatment. In some cases, the little *flaps* themselves are treated; this is just as effective and does not cause as much discomfort as might be imagined.

Due to their rubbery nature, it is sometimes difficult to pierce the tags and stalks satisfactorily, and the needle goes right through. (Skin tags do

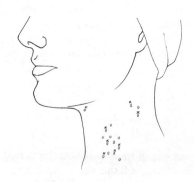

TEAR-DROP SKIN TAGS TREATMENT
STAGE 1

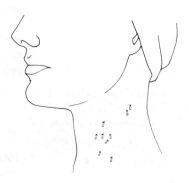

TEAR-DROP SKIN TAGS TREATMENT
STAGE 2

not normally have a good blood supply, and so this procedure is quite bearable for the client.) This does not, in fact, prevent the application from being accomplished effectively. Although the greatest intensity of current is at the tip of the needle, the current is carried along the length of the needle, and *wherever* the current meets the resistance of skin tissues along its length, it will agitate the tissues and effect a cautery. For this reason, it is necessary to remove the skin debris which has burnt on to the needle during the application, otherwise the current will be deflected from its true task and the power of the current will be diminished. (Another point to bear in mind here is that the adhering skin smells unpleasant.) The skin attached to the needle should be removed gently with the cotton-wool, dampened with lotion and held between the prongs of tweezers or by the fingers. If really firmly attached, the skin debris can be removed by drawing the tweezers slowly up the length of the needle—naturally, with the current turned off for safety. A rigid needle is essential for treating skin tags, and it must have a really fine point for accurate work.

The aftercare routine for skin tags is the same as that described for fibromas, using drying, medicated powder to speed desiccation and leaving the area undisturbed until the tags drop off. Because it is an area where friction commonly occurs, any scabs which form do tend to be rubbed off, but no harm seems to come from this and results of treatment are normally excellent. If the tags are positioned very close together, then they must be treated in a chequered fashion to avoid converging heat reactions and bad healing.

Charges for removal of skin tags and raised fibromas depend largely on the nature of the individual problem. If the condition is a single, pedunculated papilloma, which may only need one or two applications, a charge can be made for the whole treatment including any follow-up application. However, if the growths are multiple, as they often are with skin tags, and the length of time to complete the treatment uncertain, it is fairer to both operator and client to charge per treatment session.

MEDICAL REFERRAL

All work which comes under the heading cosmetic electrology can be varied in its results, especially work on fibrous growths, and much depends on the operator's ability and judgement. As has been noted earlier, small growths respond well to this form of treatment, while larger growths are better treated medically, and it is in the best interests of the client that she is advised of this fact. The electrologist should never, on her own account, treat growths or fibrous lumps growing in delicate areas such as close to the eyes or on the eyelid itself, however tiny. If the client wishes to have them treated she should be advised to consult a doctor and have them removed in a hospital situation. There will be instances, of course, where the electrologist herself will be asked by the doctor to undertake the work in the hospital, if her work has previously been noticed and approved by the medical profession. In the hospital, the operator has access not only to medical skill and knowledge to aid her techniques and guide her, but can, if necessary, complete her work under a local anaesthetic administered by the medical staff.

Conditions which fall into this category include ingrowing eyelashes, cysts on eyelids, hairs in pigmented moles, superfluous hair on children, and hair growing on the base of the spine (such as is found in spina bifida conditions).

In the course of their work, electrologists will find themselves presented with many conditions far beyond the scope and field of reference of minor cosmetic electrology. The clients may wish to have these problems resolved, and feel that the electrologist is the ideal person to help. Often the imperfection is of no medical interest and does not limit or affect the individual's health in any way, and as no help can be obtained through medical channels or the client is too embarrassed to bother medical staff about what she feels will be considered a trivial matter, she turns to the electrologist for help and guidance.

Thus, a tremendous responsibility is placed on the operator for the client's well-being, and she must face it sensibly, seeking medical assistance or suggesting that clients consult their own doctors where it seems desirable. Sometimes the client must be persuaded to live with an imperfection if it cannot be treated or would be worsened by treatment. Then, camouflage measures can be suggested: the operator can either give advice herself if she is qualified in these techniques, or can seek the help of a camouflage specialist or make-up artist.

Many imperfections can, of course, be treated with excellent results. The operator must recognize, however, when treatment should not be given, either because the condition will not benefit from treatment, or because good results cannot be guaranteed owing to her own lack of experience. It is sensible for an inexperienced operator not to take a chance on obtaining a good result, but rather to decline treatment, not only for the client's good but also for the sake of her own status and reputation.

Chapter 8

Business Practice

The electrologist's first priority has been to master the skills of her trade and obtain the qualifications which give her the right to work. Once this has been achieved, the next step, and a very vital one, is to develop a full and flourishing business practice. The essential factor here, whichever method of working is decided upon (whether being self-employed in private practice or working for an organization or private clinic) is the need to build up a regular clientele. Everywhere in the world there exists a need for the electrologist's skills, and usually all that is required to start off in business is to let the public know that you are there. This can be done through advertising or other public relations methods as well as by introductions to professional practitioners working in the allied fields of medicine, health and beauty therapy. Upon this initial base, personal recommendations then build the business clientele.

Treatment organization has already been examined (see Chapter 4) and all that remains now is to consider the various methods of work from among which the newly qualified electrologist will select the one most suited to her own experience and personal circumstances.

METHODS OF WORK

There are several ways in which the newly qualified operator can begin her career in electrology. She can work for others, while gaining experience, or work for herself, either in partnership with related beauty therapy or medical services, or entirely self-employed, running her own business. There are advantages to each of these situations. Younger operators may well prefer working among other professionals at first, enjoying their company and benefiting from the opportunity to learn from them and extend their experience. The freedom from book-keeping, handling cash, stock-keeping and other business organization procedures is also an advantage in the early stages of gaining experience, allowing full concentration to be given to acquiring practical skills and improving technique. Assuming one responsibility at a time is very much to be recommended when endeavouring to build a satisfied clientele and a successful practice.

Department Store Electrologist

The electrologist working in a department store operates in a cubicle, usually positioned close to the fashion department or hair and beauty salon. She may be employed either directly by the store or by a clinic group operating a chain of cubicles on a franchise basis. In either case, the operator's income is assured, and she has security of employment. Such operators are usually paid on a commission basis. The most common arrangement is for a basic wage to be provided, which must be covered by the practice, after which the operator receives a commission for each client treated. Many companies prefer to pay a relatively low basic wage and a high rate of commission because this encourages the operator to build up her clientele. This is a good system where a large number of potential clients are available, such as in a store, and the electrology service is well advertised and promoted by the store or parent company. All companies have slightly different commission schemes, and as these can make a tremendous difference to overall income, the operator should examine them carefully when choosing employment.

Working in a department store clinic carries a number of advantages. As there are many people

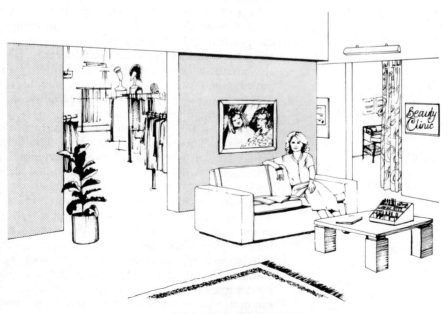

STORE ELECTROLOGIST

visiting the location to shop, it is easy to build up a good clientele and to be kept fully occupied, thus earning an excellent income. The costs and organization of advertising are borne by the store or parent organization, although the operator may well be involved in in-store promotions to inform the public of the service available. And yet, in many ways, working in a store clinic is very similar to being in private practice, without the overall responsibility for the business. Naturally, as the investment in equipment, facilities, advertising and so on has been the parent company's, so it will receive the greatest return from the epilation treatment cubicle. The risks belong to the company as well as the rewards—if the electrologist has not been selected wisely, if she is not well trained, the business will not flourish, and the cubicle could run at a loss and not even cover the rent and the overheads.

The organization of treatment appointments is normally directly controlled by the operator, although payments for treatment may possibly be made to a cashier or receptionist in the hairdressing or beauty departments to save the operator's time. Working in this way improves organizational abilities, as the operator has to be able to work quickly and efficiently and work within the strict time limits. This can be difficult at first, but practice soon corrects the slowness of a newly qualified electrologist, and it is not a point to be anxious about.

Records of clients and their appointments have to be kept to ensure both the smooth running of the practice and efficient treatment organization, as we have already observed (see Chapter 4). This also acts as a check on the size and flow of the business and provides a safeguard, should any dispute arise regarding the cubicle's earnings, and, therefore, the operator's income.

As far as the work itself is concerned, the operator is in every way her own boss. This helps her to develop a very sound level of technique in her practial work and good organizational abilities. The hours of business are normally very reasonable, matching those of the store, and the working environment most congenial. Most stores offer those working in their shops the benefit of purchase discounts on goods and the convenience of subsidized meals in staff restaurants. In addition, fitting shopping into the working day is also made easier, an especially important point for married women or working mothers to bear in mind.

Electrology Clinic Chain

There are several large companies operating clinics in cities and towns all over the UK, and in a few cases their business encompasses several countries. This considerably increases the opportunities for travel in an electrology career and improves job prospects for the young trainee.

The clinics may be fairly small, having only one or two operators, or be quite large, depending on whether they are situated in a small town or a big city. They are normally very efficiently run, thus enabling the electrologist to concentrate on performing her work to the best of her ability. Some of these clinics may be treatment areas in department stores, where the parent company operates the franchise system of offering the service. Employment and income are assured, and the opportunity exists of working for the same company in other parts of the country.

Once again, it is natural that the company providing the employment will receive the major share of the operator's takings from her practice. However, the wage paid is usually fair, and can be supplemented by commissions as clients grow in number. In an established clinic, a new operator must, of course, build up her own clientele and not expect to take them over from the other operators at the expense of their commission.

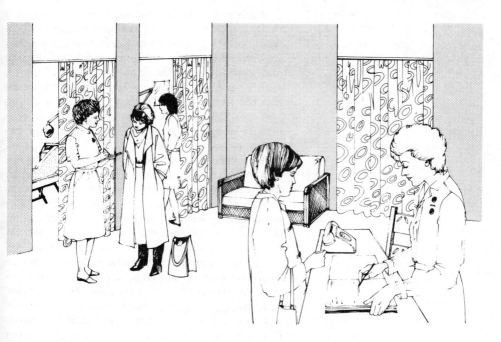

CLINIC CHAIN

However, often a new member of staff is employed to replace someone who has left, or because there is more work than the practice can handle, and so part of the new member's clientele is ready-made. If the parent company decides to open a branch in a new location, it will already have investigated the business potential before embarking on the venture. Thus, in all ways, this method of employment offers security, provided that the operator is competent and willing to work hard.

The operator may also be expected to do shift work to fit in the clients' requirements. Under a shift system, the electrologist's working week will include a combination of mornings, afternoons and evenings with the occasional weekend completely free, or days off during the week, by rotation, all members of the staff sharing the unpopular working hours. This makes for a more varied work pattern which many operators prefer. The shift system is more common in bigger towns and cities, where a large proportion of the clients work and can only come for treatment outside their own working hours. So, the service has to be provided when it is needed, and early appointments, lunch-time and evening work are all part of this system.

Private Practice

Starting a private practice from scratch is a challenge that carries all the advantages and rewards of being self-employed, but a young operator would be well advised to bear in mind some of the pitfalls and difficulties before embarking on such a venture. Setting up a new practice means that the clientele must be built up from nothing; however, once this has been successfully accomplished, the rewards for personal effort and endeavour can be excellent.

The expenditure needed to start a practice is not vast, but the long-term commitment of taking on the overheads of the business is a consideration and needs to be thought about very seriously. The initial costs include the purchase or rental of premises and any necessary alterations or decoration, as well as the purchase of equipment and materials. Running costs include the rent and/or rates, telephone, gas and electricity charges, as well as payments for materials and supplies, advertising, insurance, maintenance, accountants and professional subscriptions—without provision for all these elements the business cannot function.

If permission can be obtained to operate the business from a private residential address, your home perhaps, these costs are reduced, but not eliminated. In most instances, electrologists wishing to set up their practice at home have to obtain planning permission from the local authorities to use the premises on a business basis. This may be difficult, especially if the area is entirely residential, with no other businesses in the locality. Approval would only be granted if inspection revealed that the small business would not change the nature of the area, cause a nuisance to neighbours, or be a traffic hazard as a result of parked cars restricting the flow of traffic. The second and third points can soon be dealt with since operators can only work on one client at a time and could provide client parking on their own premises. Most applications, however, are refused on the grounds that change of use can alter a quiet residential area into a potential business location. The small, one-person enterprise is seen as setting a precedent and opening up the possibility of future applications from neighbouring homes, until quickly the area becomes a business location, rather than a residential one. The need for restriction can readily be understood. Nevertheless, some operators are lucky and gain approval to run their business from home. Once the licence to trade has been granted, the business is subject to normal trading laws, which determine hours of opening and dictate standards of qualification and hygiene. This guards against unqualified operators being able to set up in business to treat unwary customers, thus protecting both the general public and the bona fide operator.

Many private electrology practices are operated from normal business premises, either independently or in conjunction with hairdressing, or beauty and health services. If the operator does work entirely on her own, then trying to answer the phone and handle the enquiries, greet clients and make appointments, while at the same time performing the electrology service, can be very difficult. It can be done, however, because many clients have repeat appointments and, at the end of each appointment, book ahead for the next one. Many long-term clients have their appointments at a regular time of the week, and in this way seldom forget them. Furthermore, operators working on their own can allot time at the changeover of clients to permit a few moments to be spent booking future appointments. Much of this, however, is work of only a few moments once clients have got into a regular routine and know what to expect.

With a small reception area where clients can wait for their appointment, plus the actual working cubicle, the electrology working unit is complete. Regular bookings soon build up, with the majority of clients coming through personal recommendations and business referrals. Clients will not be long arriving if medical staff, nursing and community care officers, beauty and hairdressing operators are all made aware of the service being offered.

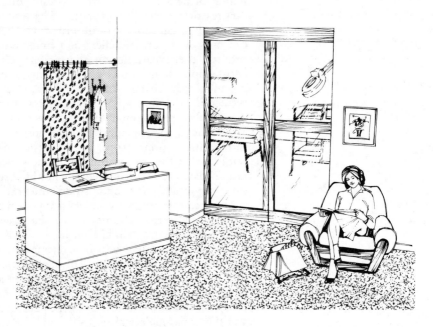

PRIVATE PRACTICE

When you run your own business, hours of work are often longer than when you are employed by someone else, and, of course, the income can be irregular. Periods of bad weather, changes in the employment or economic situation, all have a direct effect on business. Because the treatment is a necessity rather than a luxury, electrology does not suffer as badly from economic recessions as other areas of the beauty industry, but, nevertheless, it still feels the effects, and, for an owner-operated practice, these effects are immediate.

In order for a business to be successful, treatment must be offered when clients are able to attend, and this results in rather unsociable hours of work, with evening and weekend appointments being a natural part of the responsibilities of the business. Any business dependent on one individual will be a tie to that individual, and this is particularly true of a service like electrology. Electrologists do tend to live their work, finding it hard to be free of it for even short periods, and for this reason, many operators prefer not to work from a combined home and business base, because then they are never away from their work and it intrudes upon personal and family life too much.

However, the rewards are good, both in financial terms and as far as job satisfaction is concerned. There can be few more satisfying fields of work than one which relieves people of disfiguring and embarrassing hair problems which can blight their lives. Taking a treatment through from start to finish and seeing the change in the client freed from the hair problem is a positive reward in itself (see Chapter 9).

Basic accounts of income, that is cash and cheques taken for treatments and expenditure, all outgoings or expenses directly connected to the cost of running the business, must be kept. This is not a difficult task, and with advice from an accountant, very simple income and expenditure records can be kept for the accountant to present to the tax authorities each year. By completing the accounts personally, the operator can both reduce costs and also keep a careful watch on the success of the business. This record of income from appointments and outgoings on business costs is also valuable if at any stage the practice is to be sold, since it indicates the value of the clientele, and the profitability of the practice. The electrologist's own salary has to be drawn from the income obtained and, naturally, is a major cost or expense against the business. With advice from their accountants, operators can determine the most advantageous method of paying their own salaries, and the level at which it should be set, depending on their personal circumstances. The very discouraging tax situation for career women who are also wives makes essential the need for detailed advice from an accountant as to the best ways of avoiding the high tax penalties which might accrue. For instance, if a husband's and wife's income is assessed jointly, an otherwise successful practice could act as a penalty to the operator's husband. It may be preferable for her to operate as a completely separate business, not drawing a salary as such as this would be tax liable, but rather paying a company dividend on profits at the end of a financial year.

One great advantage of private practice is the chance it offers to take charge of one's own life—to be able to determine how much work one wishes to undertake, to decide when to work and when not to work. Most operators find that within a very short time they have more work than they can handle, but they always have the choice, and can put work or home first according to personal wishes. This ability to work part-time only if desired, makes electrology a very flexible profession and ideal for working mothers. A practice may perhaps be operated by two trained electrologists, both having their own clients, and working different times of the day or week to meet the demands of the business.

Last, but by no means least, personally to reap the benefits of the work put in is very pleasant, even if it has meant an investment in terms of equipment, facilities and business organization. The responsibility is rewarded in many ways for the private practitioner, and that is why a large percentage of qualified electrologists prefer to work in this way.

Part-time Hospital Electrologist

An interesting aspect of electrology for the self-employed operator is the chance to offer epilation to a local hospital on a part-time basis, perhaps one session (three to four hours) a month.

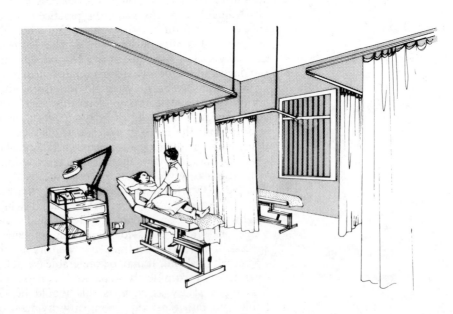

HOSPITAL ELECTROLOGIST

Payment is modest, or often non-existent, but the work is most interesting and very worthwhile, and extends the operator's experience and range of conditions. With medical backing, most unusual conditions can be treated, including hair growth relating to systemic conditions, diabetes, thyroid abnormalities, hormonal imbalance, sexual deviation (transsexual or sex-change patients), or sexual abnormality caused by endocrine malfunction (virilism). Imperfections such as hairs in moles, hairs on large growths, or hairs on children can be dealt with under local anaesthetic and ingrowing hairs and skin tags on eyelids can be treated with medical assistance. Work on clients with excessive hair problems can be completed with the advantage of sterile surroundings and rigorous attention to their overall health to aid healing and skin recovery.

Many hospital patients would be unsuitable for treatment in a general clinic practice, either because their problem is too severe or because they would be embarrassed to receive treatment outside a medical situation. In addition, for many of these patients, the cost of professional epilation on a commercial basis would be beyond their means, especially the elderly and the very young sufferers. Nevertheless, a proportion of patients, who have the time and money, will desire to obtain additional treatment beyond that which they have received in the hospital and may seek this from the electrologist in her private capacity. It would, however, be unethical for her to actively promote her private practice among patients while she is working in the hospital on a medical basis.

SITING AND LAYOUT OF AN ELECTROLOGY CLINIC

Siting

When a new practice is to be set up, the location of the premises must be viewed initially in terms of gaining clients. Once clients have got to know a clinic, then if their need is great enough and no alternatives exist, they will find their way there even if it is inconveniently situated. However, starting a new business provides one with the opportunity of trying to obtain the best site for the practice—accessible, close to transportation facilities, while also able to take advantage of a passing trade of potential clients. Naturally, however, the more 'convenient' the premises are, the higher will be the rent for the space.

Easy access is important, especially for elderly clients who may have to rely on public transport. If the practice is in a small town, adequate parking facilities must be provided, as most of the clients will travel by car; access to a nearby multi-storey or public car park is a real asset. Since most appointments are of such short duration, clients welcome the opportunity to combine the epilation treatment with another task or grooming service, and, for this reason, the combination of an independent practice operating alongside another service can prove very beneficial. Clients then only have to park once and can undertake several tasks in the one visit, combining hairdressing, beauty therapy or chiropody with their epilation appointment. The growth of department store cubicles for electrology, which enables clients to combine business with pleasure, would seem to confirm this point.

So, the practice needs to be central, convenient to transport and have good parking nearby. Ideally it should also not be too difficult to find and be on ground level, although first floor premises are more common, as they prove to be more available and less expensive. If the clinic is rather tucked away or operates in a group practice, it should be well marked, and its exact location should be stressed in advertising and during telephone enquiries from prospective clients.

A new trend in many parts of the world is to locate the practice in a shopping centre, usually in

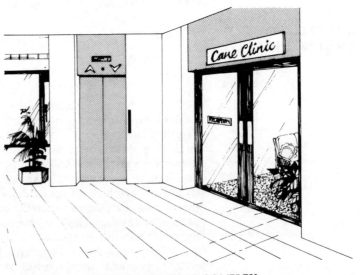

CLINIC IN SHOPPING COMPLEX

the office accommodation above the shopping complex, among a wide range of business services. This has the advantage of offering public parking and a wide range of shopping facilities, while providing a quiet and pleasant atmosphere for work. In addition to medical practitioners, opticians, beauty therapists and dentists, the electrologist is finding many advantages in siting her business in this type of location. The changing role of the shopping centre in providing a place of entertainment and leisure, as well as supplying shopping needs and banking facilities, makes it a social centre which attracts a wide population— the electrologist's clients coming from all walks of life.

Within the shopping complex, the business will have little passing trade and so will, initially, have to devote more money to advertising to make the public aware of the service. Since a discreet nameplate may be all that informs the client that a practice is in being, personal recommendations are vital in building up trade, and public relations work is essential for business success.

Layout

Only a very small area is required to operate an epilation service, simply a treatment area or cubicle containing the couch and trolley, plus the magnifier, epilation machine and commodities for treatment. The working position needs good light and should ideally be positioned close to a window; working in natural daylight is much less tiring than working under artificial light, and makes it possible for far longer periods of very exacting and concentrated work to be performed in comfort and without eyestrain.

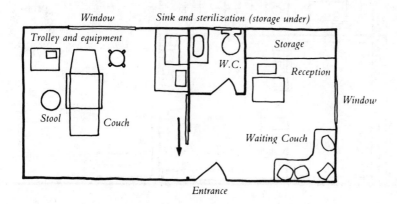

PRIVATE PRACTICE LAYOUT

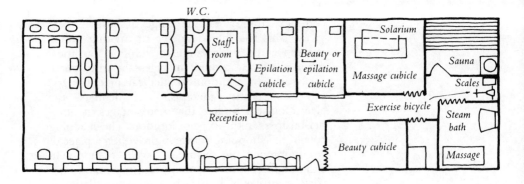

HAIR/BEAUTY THERAPY/EPILATION LAYOUT

An electrology clinic may have its own reception and waiting areas, or share them if it operates in conjunction with other services. In an owner-operated practice, only a small reception area is required as the practitioner can only work on one person at a time, and there is little overlap of clients. A clinic chain, employing several operators, however, will need a waiting and reception area in proportion to the number of treatment units or cubicles. The appointment bookings, cash handling and client reception are all then taken care of by a receptionist.

If the practice is located in a private home or small office premises, two small rooms can be set aside as a reception and waiting room and a treatment room, or, if there are insufficient rooms to make this possible, the available space can be

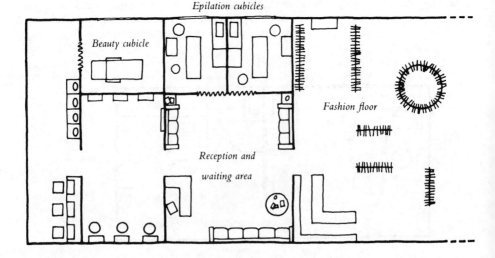

DEPARTMENT STORE LAYOUT

divided up to provide a working and a waiting area, separated by curtains, screens or partitions. It is also possible for an operator in her own business to pace treatments so that clients do not overlap at all, but simply come directly to the treatment room as they arrive, eliminating the need for a real waiting area.

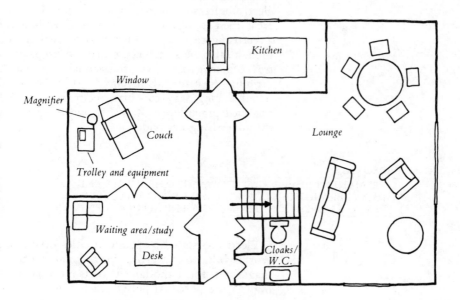

HOME EPILATION LAYOUT

DEVELOPING A PRACTICE

When starting in professional practice, the electrologist has to set out in a determined way to build up a clientele sufficient to sustain her business. As epilation treatments are well spaced, usually with two or three weeks at least between each appointment, many clients are needed to fill the operator's week. Because of this rotating nature of attendance, and the fact that clients do *complete* their courses of treatment and are then lost to the practice, new clients have to be sought at all times.

There are two main ways in which this can be accomplished: through advertising, which usually costs money and is paid for by the business, and through public relations and publicity measures, which cost time but not normally money.

Advertising

Advertising acts to inform the public of the service and is a necessary part of any business venture. For an electrology practice, it can take the form of small newspaper advertisements, repeated regularly in the personal column of the paper. This appears to work well for many practitioners, who keep an advertisement running in their local daily or weekly paper at all times. This reaches the local people in the area who will be within travelling distance of the practice. If only one electrologist is in business in a widespread country area, then it may be well worth extending this advertising to take in other nearby districts and their local papers, as clients may be prepared to travel further to receive professional help. This is certainly the case with advanced work: clients will travel a long way to obtain help from a well-qualified practitioner. It is then worth spreading the advertising net wider.

PERSONAL

PERMANENT REMOVAL OF UNWANTED HAIR. SAFE AND PAIN FREE METHOD. CONSULT MRS GREEN. DIPLOMA IN REMEDIAL EPILATION. TEL. 743–0214. FOR APPOINTMENT.

Electrologists who operate in cities may find it worthwhile to advertise in popular women's magazines, for, although the costs are very much higher, the potential public reached is immense, and, where a practice must compete for its clients, then the costs are justified.   For a qualified operator belonging to a professional association or institute of electrology, an opportunity often exists to link in with a national advertising compaign (perhaps in a women's magazine), organized through the national office. The cost of this form of promotion may be borne by the annual subscriptions to the organization, or members may be asked to contribute to the scheme. With this form of advertising, it is the association or institute, and the high standard of professional work for which it stands, that is being promoted. Interested readers of the advertisement are asked to write in for further information about electrology, which they receive together with the address and telephone number of the nearest association or institute member. This system works very well as an information service, and in fact most professional electrology associations have a member's directory or list from which a potential client can obtain the name and address of a member who can help her with her problem.

Advertising in the *Yellow Pages* of the telephone directory appears to be effective in many cases,

Unwanted Hair?

   Solve the Problem for EVER.

For a SAFE and Permanent ANSWER
to your HAIR PROBLEM
CONSULT
Your Local Institute of Electrolysis member.

MRS B. SMITHE D.R.E.

Tel. 43-62-0919—Clinic-42
(CRN · Freemont & Brant)   Freemont

and here full use should be made of the qualifications and letters which are inserted after the business name to denote the level of training completed. Clients do have a genuine anxiety over the pain, marking or permanent skin damage caused by permanent hair removal, and indicating the qualifications which the operator has obtained goes a long way to allay these fears. Many operators stress their professional membership when using this form of advertising, for example, 'Your Local Institute of Electrolysis Member, Mrs B. Smithe, D.R.E. (Diploma in Remedial Epilation) ... (plus details of the business address and telephone number).' The qualification had been hard won, so it is something to be proud of and to use in building up a professional practice.

Publicity and Public-relations Work

Publicity and public-relations exercises are probably the most effective ways of attracting clients to a new business, and time must be spent on these aspects in the early days. Later, when the business has become known and a reputation for good work has been established, personal recommendations from clients will play the largest part in helping to keep the operator busy. Initially, however, informing the public and related trades and professions—hairdressing, beauty therapy, chiropody, medical, ophthalmic and other health-linked agencies—of the service and gaining their support is vital to success, and there are a number of ways in which this can be achieved.

MUTUAL EXCHANGE OF INFORMATION

Building a good business relationship with associated fields is possibly the single most effective way of developing a successful practice. By doing this, practitioners are able to help each other, not only by simple advertising measures such as displaying each other's business cards in their reception areas, but also by giving personal recommendations to their own clients about other services when asked for information or advice.

CONTACT WITH PROMINENT PEOPLE

Contact with individuals holding prominent positions in the local community is also useful and can result in a lot of new business. Chairwomen of civic groups, leaders of voluntary service organizations, Red Cross organizers and representatives of the welfare services, all have contact with a large number of potential clients and can inform them of the service that is available. One way of acquainting these influential people with the service is to invite them to view the facilities and meet the operator, either at a personal visit or at an open evening. Most of them will recognize the value that a service of this kind could be to the community, and will pass on the information to individuals whom they know would benefit from it. Once a client, who is in contact with a large group of women, either in a paid or voluntary capacity, has been gained, she will be instrumental in bringing more clients to the practice.

PUBLIC LECTURES

Any opportunity to talk about the work of the electrologist should be eagerly accepted, whether it is at a meeting of the Mothers' Union or Women's Institute, young wives' organization or old people's gathering. There are potential clients in every group, and it is a wonderful chance to describe the work and inform the audience of the help that is available. It also provides an occasion to dispel a few fears and anxieties that may be holding people back from seeking help. New methods, the latest techniques and the lack of scarring can all be discussed in an informal, but knowledgeable way.

HOSPITAL WORK

Working in the local hospital, perhaps even just one session a month, can be a very valuable way of building up a practice. The operator will become known among the patients, and those who can afford her services may well seek help from her in a private capacity, either to speed up the treatment which they are currently undertaking or to help them with some other condition. As has already been observed, however, the electrologist must on no account *solicit* clients from among her hospital patients.

Referrals by doctors make up a large percentage of some electrologists' work, and are, therefore, very important to their business. Whether these referrals occur depends to a considerable extent on the relationship created with local medical staff. If the local doctors, and their staff are informed about the operator's field of work and are sympathetic to the needs of the patients in this respect, then recommendations will be forthcoming. Patients will no longer be advised to remove unwanted hair by shaving or other temporary methods, as was the case in the past and, in some instances, is still the case today.

It is worth taking the time to visit local doctors personally, at a time convenient to them, to explain the qualifications held, the service that will be offered and the kind of clients that can be helped. Working in co-operation with the medical profession to help in the overall process of patient care is one of the most gratifying aspects of professional electrology. The more advanced the work of the clinic practice becomes, the more the operator will need medical guidance and advice to ensure that clients receive the best possible care. It is a far more satisfactory and courteous arrangement to see that the electrologist and her work are known to a doctor *before* his or her patients start seeking medical approval for treatment of various conditions: the doctor will naturally want to know *what* the treatment is he or she is recommending or approving for a patient, and *by whom* it is to be performed. Approval may well not be given without this knowledge.

All these aspects of public relations and promotional work also serve to inform the general public of the value and relevance of professional electrology and the service it can offer. This is how the reputation of the profession and, thereby, the status of its practitioners grows. To work in a well-respected profession is very rewarding and provides excellent job satisfaction to lighten the load of the work.

Insurance

It is essential, when operating a business practice involving members of the public, that professional and business insurance is properly organized. It should be set up in such a way that *all* risks are covered, to safeguard both the operator and the client.

The actual business premises and its contents must, of course, be insured against the event of fire, damage or theft. Less obvious is the need to protect the business and the operator against claims from customers, as a result of either personal injury sustained while on the premises, or damage caused by the epilation application itself. Many well-qualified operators are able to obtain very competitive insurance rates for personal indemnity through their professional associations. These 'blanket' schemes of insurance for members reflect the high standard of training and examination necessary to obtain membership of the association, and indicate that the association and its members are held in esteem by the insurance companies, and are, therefore, classed as a low risk. Since, few, if any claims have ever been lodged against association members, they benefit from a really low rate of personal coverage. It can be very difficult to obtain personal insurance in the electrology business at realistic rates on an *individual* basis, since, in any area of work concerning the client's appearance, there is always an element of risk involved. Large claims for loss of appearance are regularly lodged against operators in the beauty and hairdressing industries, making the industry as a whole a high risk area in the eyes of the insurance companies. In the UK, claims of this kind are rare, but this is mainly due to the high standard of training, and consumer awareness.

In an owner-operated business, it is also a good idea to insure against inability to work through injury, accidents or illness, since the entire income of the business depends upon the individual's capacity to work. Like all insurance, this is a direct cost against the business, and a very necessary and justified expense.

LEGAL REQUIREMENTS

As has been seen, there are specific legal requirements which have to be met before setting up business as a sole trader or practitioner. These requirements will vary somewhat in different areas of the world, but will have basic similarities. It is wise to determine from the local authorities what requirements there are regarding permission to trade—planning regulations for the location of the business, the licensing regulations and any other matters which must be complied with before the business can be started. In some countries, 'red tape' is kept to a minimum, while in others it seems to be set up solely to discourage even the most determined business venture. This is mainly due to the greater risk existing in some countries from unqualified operators (in any field, not only electrology) and for the use of premises for purposes other than those for which they are intended. If allowed to go unregulated, these, and many other abuses of the system, would work against both the public's interests and those of the qualified operator trying to offer a good service.

In countries where there is a good consumer awareness and epilation is well-known, only qualified operators feel able to set up in business. Clients know that they should attend only a qualified specialist, and many media sources (such as magazines, newspapers, television) help them to find that professional help. Where the professional electrology associations work in co-operation with medical and official government bodies, clients feel secure in the knowledge that operators have official recognition and work under stringent controls.

However, achieving this recognition and status takes time, and in countries where the industry is new, other more restrictive measures have to be used to protect the consumer. Licensing of qualified operators and their premises is one way to do this; the operator must meet the official requirements for length and level of training before being granted permission to work. Outside Europe, the official standards or requirements will vary tremendously. In certain countries, electrology is a medical responsibility, and is not regarded as a health-*related* field at all. In other countries, electrology is performed by non-medical operators, but comes directly under the jurisdiction of the medical authorities and is controlled by them. Electrologists must meet the same requirements as practitioners in other health-related fields such as chiropody, acupuncture, etc. Therefore, electrologists embarking on a business venture, especially in a country other than the one in which training was undertaken, should acquaint themselves with all the regulations in case their qualifications are not accepted by a reciprocal agreement.

Most countries have strong professional associations or institutes which, through the hard work of their committees over many years, have forged a good relationship with the medical profession. Joining a professional organization is normally a very supportive element for an independent practitioner, and, naturally, the organization relies for its strength on the numbers of members it can attain.

BENEFITS OF MEMBERSHIP OF PROFESSIONAL ELECTROLOGY ORGANIZATIONS

Membership of professional bodies provides a means of keeping up to date with new techniques, equipment and information, through periodic meetings, news bulletins and social gatherings of members. It promotes a high standard of practical and theoretical knowledge and maintains a professional status for its members. It builds a good relationship with the medical profession and other well-known organizations, thus creating a good working atmosphere based on mutual trust and respect.

Insurance for professional work is available, either linked with annual membership or offered at preferential rates.

Most organizations have a membership list or a national register of qualified operators, listing their qualifications and the range of treatments they offer. These lists are available to the general public, either by private or press enquiries, or through public libraries, etc. This practice of joining the larger organizations is growing as younger operators see the advantages of gaining professional status, and it is hoped this will eventually lead to government recognition of the need for full registration to safeguard the public from untrained practitioners.

ELECTROLOGY TRAINING

There are several ways to obtain a training in electrology, either independently or in association with beauty therapy. Training may be obtained in private schools by payment of a fee, or in technical colleges through government-funded courses. Major companies may also offer training in the field, but in this case the operator will have to sign a contract agreeing to work for the company for a set period after training has been completed to compensate the company for the cost of training.

There are several institutes and associations which offer **training in epilation exclusively**. This training may be through registered tutors in private practice, for which a fee is paid, or in schools or colleges, with the organization stipulating the training requirements. Training in private practice lasts six months to one year and prepares students for the final examinations of the major associations. The schools also work closely with the examining bodies to ensure that students receive the necessary level of theoretical and practical knowledge to be successful in their exams. Practical tuition is normally of at least two hundred hours' duration, and theoretical studies a minimum of forty hours. These requirements are designed to meet the minimum standards laid down by the licensing authorities in countries where licensing controls exist. They are also the accepted levels agreed by the major training bodies as necessary to achieve competence in the work.

Many younger students undertake **electrology training in conjunction with beauty therapy courses**, and in this way increase their employment potential. In professional practice, they will divide their time between beauty therapy work and electrology, and many find this less tiring, both on the eyes and the nerves. College courses must still include the same number of hours of practical electrology tuition as if the electrology training were undertaken independently—there is no way to short-cut gaining the practical skills. Although electrology requires a more advanced knowledge in some areas, the theoretical aspects of electrology and beauty therapy are similar in many aspects. The theory subjects are, therefore, co-ordinated to save time, and, for this reason, colleges seldom offer training for electrology alone, but nearly always as part of a full therapy course.

Colleges in major centres such as London do sometimes offer **part-time training** to students who already hold some other qualification, for example nursing, beauty therapy or physiotherapy certificates, and want to extend or alter their field of work.

Professional Bodies—Courses and Awards

INSTITUTE OF ELECTROLYSIS

Diploma in Remedial Epilation (DRE)

The Institute offers associate or full membership to its potential students, depending on their age and general background. The associate member will normally attempt to gain full membership when her age and circumstances become acceptable to the Institute's Council. The main qualification, the Diploma in Remedial Epilation (DRE), is normally taught on an individual basis by a registered tutor within a clinic situation. The diploma course covers all aspects of skin and hair histology, and demands an extremely high standard of operating technique in practical epilation. Training is normally full-time, of at least six hundred hours, including no less than three hundred hours of practical work, and is on a private basis, through tutors, and entry to the Institute's membership is by examination only. Operators working within the industry are also eligible to sit for the diploma examination, if they have been in continuous practice for a period of at least two years.

BRITISH ASSOCIATION OF ELECTROLYSISTS

The Association provides a professional organization for trained electrologists, and its aims are to elevate the profession as a whole, to promote their interests and efficiency by the observance of a strict system of training and examination for all those seeking admission to membership and entering the profession.

Candidates may apply for membership after they have completed the required syllabus of training, including a minimum of two hundred hours of practical epilation, over a period of not less than six months after reaching a competent stage. Students must have reached the age of eighteen years before the start of their course. Training is based on the official syllabus of the British Association of Electrolysists, and students can train either with private tutors or at courses offered at colleges of higher education or colleges of technology throughout the UK.

AMERICAN ELECTROLYSIS ASSOCIATION

The American Electrolysis Association was incorporated in 1958 as a non-profit-making educational organization for increasing knowledge in the field of electrology, and to establish closer relationship between electrologists throughout the USA, the UK and Europe. The organization has as its purpose the improvement of ethics, standards and education in the electrolysis profession, and works for the improvement of relations between the profession, allied professions, and the general public.

The Association was also organized in order to assist all efforts for the promotion of better standards through state legislation, establishing rules and regulations which call for higher educational and social standards, the inclusion of the basic sciences in schools and teachers' curricula throughout the USA.

The Association acts as a source of reference and information to its members, and through news letters, meetings at state level and bi-annual national conferences, keeps its members informed of all new advances and developments relating to professional electrology.

CITY AND GUILDS OF LONDON INSTITUTE

City and Guilds Beauty Therapist's Certificate 761

The two-year, full-time course leading up to this certificate covers all aspects of facial and body treatments, and is provided by selected colleges throughout the UK. Students must be at least eighteen years old and have a minimum academic qualification of three O level GCE subjects. Due to the competition for places, colleges can be very selective in their choice of applicant, and may demand a higher level of GCE passes than the minimum requirement. Tuition is divided between theoretical and practical aspects of therapy, permitting confidence to develop in client handling and practical techniques. The longer period of training makes this an ideal course for the younger woman, and allows skills to become established under the guidance of an experienced lecturer.

City and Guilds Certificate in Electrical Epilation 761–3

Run in conjunction with the Beauty Therapist's Certificate, the training covers both theoretical and practical aspects of permanent hair removal by electrical methods. Students are given the opportunity to obtain clinical practice, and can build up knowledge of individual case histories of clients during the training period. A minimum of two hundred hours of practical epilation application is the requirement specified by the examination board before students may enter for the final examinations. So, this qualification denotes a very high standard of electrology skill and knowledge.

INTERNATIONAL HEALTH AND BEAUTY COUNCIL NATIONAL HEALTH AND BEAUTY COUNCIL (UK)

The International Beauty Therapist's Diploma

This course is widely available, on a one- or two-year basis, at further education colleges, private schools and training establishments. The course covers all aspects of salon work, facial and body treatments, figure improvement and cosmetic applications, plus background theory relating to the practical subjects.

Some colleges in the UK offer a two-year course combining the International Beauty Therapist's Diploma and the City and Guilds Beauty Therapist's Certificate. In this way, students benefit from the wide range of subjects covered, while establishing practical skills through salon sessions and client handling. Students are encouraged to undertake training in related subjects, such as electrology and remedial camouflage, during the two-year training period, to enhance their career prospects and extend their experience of remedial work.

More frequently, the diploma is offered independently as a one-year course, and it attracts a reasonable proportion of more mature applicants, who may have previous experience in nursing, commerce or cosmetic work.

The International Beauty Therapist's Diploma is one of the best-known and respected therapy qualifications available around the world.

The Beauty Specialist's Diploma

The Beauty Specialist's Diploma covers all aspects of facial therapy, grooming treatments and arm and leg applications. It is often a forerunner to full therapy training, as the demand is increasingly to offer a full service requiring all-round qualifications. The Beauty Specialist's course is available on a one-year basis in the college situation, often followed by a further period of body-work training. It is available in commercial schools and private training establishments, on a full- or part-time basis, and provides a nationally recognized qualification for full facial work. The course covers practical and theoretical aspects of facial therapy, cosmetic and physical science and business organization.

The Certificate in Epilation

This certificate is usually offered in conjunction with full-time therapy courses to provide additional basic qualifications in electrology and depilatory treatments.

The Diploma in Advanced Electrology

The course covers advanced techniques of electrology, and is a progression from the Certificate in Epilation. Students must possess the certificate level of qualification, or be exempted by reason of an alternative professional qualification, before they can start training at the advanced level. The course covers specialized aspects of permanent hair removal and minor cosmetic electrology (treatment of dilated capillaries, skin tags, etc.). A very high standard of practical and theoretical knowledge is required for successful completion of the course. Qualification is by examination only, covering both practical work and theoretical knowledge of anatomy, electrophysics and the functions of the endocrine system.

Remedial Camouflage Diploma

This qualification covers all the techniques using cosmetic means to camouflage severe skin blemishes, scars and pigmentation abnormalities. Also included is the cosmetic, post-operative treatment of plastic surgery patients. Entry to training is restricted to those who already possess a basic beauty qualification in facial therapy, or who have considerable clinical experience or are concurrently training for an IHBC qualification (Beauty Specialist's Diploma or International Beauty Therapist's Diploma).

LE COMITÉ INTERNATIONALE D'ESTHÉTIQUES ET DE COSMETOLOGY (CIDESCO)

The International CIDESCO Diploma has been recognized for over thirty years and held in esteem in more than twenty-seven countries around the world. The CIDESCO training is uniform in all countries, being of at least one year's duration, plus a probationary period of six months, before the full diploma is granted. Training *must* be of at least twelve hundred hours' duration, for practical and theoretical work, and covers facial and body therapy, cosmetic applications, treatment of the hands and feet and waxing therapy. Study options are also offered to extend the student's range of experience, and these can be tailored to the student's natural interests and area of chosen work. The study options include electrical epilation, care of the breasts, scalp treatments, specialized massage, care of the body and rhythmical movement.

Students must be at least eighteen years old before they sit their final examinations, although many CIDESCO students are older than this minimum, as maturity of outlook is a very desirable asset for a therapist. Students are also expected to have a sound educational background, so that they may benefit from the training undertaken. With the courses offered in the UK, and examined by the Confederation of Beauty Therapy and Cosmetology, the entry requirements are for a minimum of three subjects at GCE O-level (or the equivalent, at the discretion of the college). Good oral and written ability in the language of the country in which the training is undertaken, plus a sound background to the science studies, are necessary. Anatomy, cosmetic science and physics are all taught as related theory on the course, to support the understanding of the practical work.

Exacting conditions for recognition as a CIDESCO training school, as far as facilities and qualification and experience of staff are concerned, ensure that a high standard of tuition is received, which will meet the international standard. After successful completion of the course, students must work in a first-class beauty centre for a further six months, after which they can apply for the full CIDESCO Diploma. This does ensure that only serious, career-minded therapists are recognized by CIDESCO.

THE CONFEDERATION OF BEAUTY THERAPY AND COSMETOLOGY

Esthéticienne Diploma Course

The Esthéticienne Diploma course covers facial and body therapy and electrology, and is organized by the British Association of Beauty Therapy and Cosmetology. It is examined by the Confederation of Beauty Therapy and Cosmetology, which is the British Board recognized by CIDESCO and permitted to offer qualification to the international CIDESCO level to students able to meet the necessary requirements.

On successful completion of the Esthéticienne Diploma course, having gained a pass rate of 65% or over in all sections of the examination, students at selected schools can continue their studies to reach the CIDESCO standard of qualification. Approval to offer the CIDESCO course is only granted to a small number of schools and educational establishments in the UK at present. It is normally offered as a one-year, full-time course in private schools and a two-year course in further education colleges. (This allows for the longer holidays given by the state schools.)

The Esthéticienne Diploma course taken independently has a minimum training period specified by the Confederation of seven to eight months in private schools and one year in the further education colleges.

Beautician Diploma Course

This qualification covers all subjects relevant to a beauty operator practising facials, manicures, make-up, waxing, eye-lash tinting, etc. The course provides three hundred hours of training.

Electrolysis Diploma Course

This course covers practical electrology and theoretical studies of anatomy and electrical science. The course requirement is for two hundred and forty hours of study.

INTERNATIONAL THERAPY EXAMINATION CENTRE (ITEC)

ITEC provides an independent examination system which is widely recognized around the English-speaking world. Qualifications are offered through registered training establishments for all levels of facial and body therapy.

Beauty Therapy Diploma

The course covers both facial and body therapy, and the related theory of anatomy, electrical science and cosmetic chemistry. Students are able to work in a pratical situation to gain clinical experience, at the same time as studying for the theory examinations.

Esthéticienne Diploma

Training covers the beauty aspects of facial therapy only and is designed to concentrate on manual and electrical therapy, with related background therapy.

Chapter 9

Case Histories

By looking at a selection of treatment case histories, it is possible to see how an epilation programme can progress to a successful conclusion. Every case has to be planned to meet the client's individual needs, but similarities in the application of the techniques will be apparent in many instances, and this knowledge can be used as the basis of planning any treatment programme.

By considering the consultation, treatment plan, treatment progression and treatment application, one can see exactly how a problem can be resolved and the relatively few hours of professional epilation actually involved.

CASE HISTORY 1: POST-MENOPAUSAL HAIR GROWTH

Consultation

A mature fifty-two-year-old client has a typical menopausal hair growth condition. The normal vellus hair has developed into superfluous growth over the last five years. There are long, horny hairs associated with the vellus hairs on the upper lip, the strongest hairs being at the corner of the mouth, while, on the chin, there are long hairs of a fine, wispy appearance associated with abnormal, very strong hairs, which are centred into two clumps, one each side of the chin. The skin texture is well balanced, not excessively dry, and considered by the client to heal easily and be unlikely to suffer allergic reactions. The client has been plucking the hairs out for many years, so the full potential of unwanted hairs will not be evident for some time (see Chapter 4).

Treatment Plan

The epilation applications are well-spaced to avoid over-treatment until skin reactions are known. The strong, evident hairs in the chin clumps and on the side lip areas are treated in a chequered manner, interspersed with work on the finer growth, to rest the client and extend her treatment capacity. Strong hairs are treated with a .004 diameter Ferrie needle, using an intensity of 2½, and adjusting the application of the current to suit the diameter of the hair and the sensitivity of the skin. Fine hairs are treated with the same needle, or a finer one (.003) if the follicles are very small, using an intensity of 1½ to avoid surface burns. The skin reaction is excellent, showing very little effect after twenty minutes of slow treatment, so a treatment programme is started.

Treatment Progression

Fortnightly appointments of twenty minutes are undertaken, with work continuing on all areas systematically. The strongest hairs which cause distress are removed first, and regrowth dealt with subsequently as it emerges. Work on the finer hairs also progresses so that fine, original hairs and the regrowth from the stronger hairs are dealt with simultaneously.

The client is advised not to pluck out any hairs, but to cut them close to the skin when she feels the necessity to remove them. In the first two months of epilation treatment, many of the previously plucked hairs emerge, and a more accurate picture of the quantity of hair present is gained and discussed with the client.

After four months, the worst stage of the treatment is over, with the strong hairs having reached a point where regrowth does not occur and finer hairs being cleared rapidly with minimal regrowth. At this stage, it is now a question of dealing with the sheer quantity of existing hair, and, as the client is keen to resolve her problem, appointments continue at fortnightly intervals. Whole areas are emerging free from hair, and regrowth is wispy. This regrowth must, however, be removed to prevent it reverting into stronger hair through internal, hormonal stimulus (see Chapter 5). The dominance of male hormones over female hormones after the menopause can cause hair growth well into old age, and the client may quite possibly need 'tidy-up' treatments for the rest of her life.

After eight months, the hair problem is almost resolved, and the current intensity used to remove the regrowth hairs is reduced. The skin is in good condition, and the enlarged pores caused by the size of the superfluous hairs have become refined and smaller. Treatment appointments become three-weekly.

One year after the first treatment, only periodic sessions are needed, as and when the lip and chin area looks rather untidy. These 'tidy-up' sessions become three-monthly, and eventually six-monthly.

Treatment Application	Total Treatment Time	
	Hours	Minutes
First 4 months, 20-minute appointments, fortnightly	2	40
Next 4 months, 20-minute appointments, fortnightly	2	40
Last 4 months, 20-minute appointments, every 3 weeks	1	40
	7	00

Plus 6-monthly tidy-up treatments, or as needed.

CASE HISTORY 2: FACIAL HAIR LINKED TO PREGNANCY

Consultation

A young mother, twenty-three years old with three small children aged four years, two-and-a-half years and nine months, has a hair problem relating to her pregnancies. The superfluous hair is a dense, blonde growth on the upper lip, fine in texture, with well-spaced, wispy hairs on the chin. The client has fair colouring and a hyper-sensitive skin which gentle cleansing during skin inspection causes to redden fiercely. The hair condition had become a small problem following the second pregnancy and had been worsened by the third pregnancy in four years. Now, the unwanted hair is sufficient to embarrass the client, and she seeks a permanent solution.

The client has no past or present history of artificial hormone medication and had not taken the Pill, and now, with her family complete, is using the 'coil' (IUD) as her method of contraception. So, the superfluous hair growth would appear to be due to a family or personal predisposition, triggered in this case by the multiple, closely spaced pregnancies and associated increased hormonal levels at these times. Medical help has been sought, and as no other cause seemed apparent, the client was advised to try epilation from a qualified electrologist. The client contacted the electrologist after reading an article on electrology in a leading women's magazine. She had written to the professional associations listed and been sent a list of members' names in her area.

Treatment Plan

The young client had periodically used a chemical depilatory to remove the unwanted hairs, often with bad skin reaction. The initial inspection reveals that the skin is fragile, sore and easily irritated, and short hairs with blunt ends are visible, following chemical, temporary removal. This skin fragility explains the extreme reaction which occurred on skin cleansing. The client is advised to get the skin into a healthier condition prior to epilation treatment to prevent bad skin reactions. A plan is devised which will resolve the problem as quickly as possible, considering the skin's sensitivity, and which will allow the client to maintain a reasonable appearance while undergoing treatment. The client is willing not to use temporary methods to remove the hair if this will speed up the whole removal process and will hide the offending hairs with make-up. Only when it is absolutely necessary will she resort to cutting them. No plucking or chemical depilatories are to be used as the skin is so sensitive.

Treatments are to be every ten days initially. The hairs being treated should be well spaced, and an insulated steel needle used on the very shallow lip hairs. The applications are given in short, fifteen minute sessions, with meticulous pre- and aftercare measures, including the use of ozone steaming to aid healing (cool-antibacterial effect). The ozone steaming is applied for five minutes prior to epilation, and ten minutes following the application. The minimum amount of current is used, in this instance an intensity of 1½, applied for a fraction of a second.

Treatment Progression

After three months the skin has settled down and fortnightly treatment sessions of twenty minutes' duration can be given, with ozone steaming only required after the application to reduce erythema. By this stage, after regular treatment at frequent, though short, sessions, the denseness of the lip hair growth is decreasing, and regrowth hair is being removed alongside original hairs. The wispy hairs on the chin have all been treated once and have not regrown.

After six months of regular treatment, the problem is almost resolved, and the client does not need to cut the offending hairs. After a thorough 'clearing up' treatment session, the skin is given a month's rest for healing and recovery. In this month, hairs will regrow, and final clearance can take place over the next few months.

After nine months (eight months of treatment, plus one rest month), the problem is almost gone, and the client can finish her programme with three-weekly sessions. Hairs have been quite stubborn in terms of the amount of regrowth, but in one year the problem is completely solved to the client's satisfaction. The predisposition to hair growth may cause future problems at later stages of life, and the client may need to seek professional assistance again.

Treatment Application	Total Treatment Time	
	Hours	Minutes
First 3 months, 15-minute appointments, at 10-day intervals	2	15
Next 3 months, 20-minute appointments, fortnightly	2	00
Next month, rest		
Next 2 months, 20-minute appointments, fortnightly	1	20
Last 3 months, 20-minute appointments, every 3 weeks	1	20
	6	55

CASE HISTORY 3: HAIR PROBLEM ASSOCIATED WITH DIABETES MELLITUS

Consultation

A young woman of Jewish extraction, suffering from diabetes mellitus, has an upper-lip hair problem, plus scattered chin and cheek hairs. She is married, twenty-seven years of age, and has one child after a very difficult pregnancy as a result of her diabetes. The client recalls becoming aware of her increased hair growth after the child's birth, possibly as a result of the increased medications taken to maintain a successful pregnancy and ensure a healthy child. The client's diabetes was diagnosed in her late teens and is now controlled by daily injections of insulin and rigid dietary controls; she has adjusted her life to her health, and in this way can cope with her busy family life. The client has suffered from a disrupted skin condition since adolescence. It is sensitive, easily irritated, slow to heal and, like many diabetic skins, prone to rashes, spots, etc. Tiredness and anxiety seem to have a direct effect on the skin's condition. The client tells of good and bad periods with both her physical, systemic condition and her skin. Medical approval has been given for the treatment.

Treatment Plan

The actual hair condition is not the main problem, and on another skin and a different client would have been classed as minor and easy to resolve. The client's systemic condition, diabetes mellitus, and its associated skin disturbance and poor healing capacity are the major obstacles to success. However, with a very flexible treatment plan, paced to the client's health, treatment can progress.

Treatment Progression

Initially, short sessions of epilation are applied, backed up with ozone steaming before and after each session. Skin reaction on the first few treatments is severe and makes long healing gaps of three to four weeks necessary. Gradually, the skin reactions become less severe as different healing measures are used to aid the healing process. On medical advice, the client uses a medicated cream to heal the skin, which can be obtained on prescription only. Insulated, steel needles are used to minimize surface reaction. It is also found that the 'high-fast' method of application reduces the erythema reaction considerably, and causes less client discomfort. This naturally means that probing has to be extremely accurate, and the current discharged for the very minimum period necessary to accomplish removal of the hair. In this case, regrowth is inevitable: although the 'high-fast' method is used, that is discharge of the current for a fraction of a second on a high intensity, rather than the low-slow method, *overall only a tiny amount of current can be used due to the sensitivity of the skin*. This amount is, in fact, far too little to destroy the growing capacity of the hair follicles. The *amount* of current is the same, but simply applied quickly rather than slowly. This, linked with the use of an insulated, steel needle and ozone steaming, makes treatment possible, if not completely satisfactory. However, the client is determined to proceed, and the appointments settle at fifteen minutes' duration, every two weeks, with original and regrowth hairs being treated together.

By eight months of reasonably regular treatment the client's skin is still standing up to the treatment and the hair problem is well on the way to being resolved. At this point, appointments are again set at three-weekly intervals to help the skin condition, since the worst of the embarrassing problem is now over. Without aggravation from plucking, chemical depilatories and so on, all used periodically prior to epilation, the skin becomes much calmer and less subject to outbreaks and irritations.

After a year and a half, including several rest periods to allow both the skin and the client to recover, the problem is almost resolved. Treatment can be finished on a monthly basis and is brought to a successful conclusion within the second year.

Treatment Application	Total Treatment Time	
	Hours	Minutes
First 4 months, 15-minute appointments, every 3 to 4 weeks	1	15
Next 4 months, 15-minute appointments, every 2 weeks	2	00
Next 4 months, 15-minute appointments, every 3 weeks	1	15
Next month, rest (break from treatment for skin/ general health)		
Next 6 months, 15-minute appointments, every 3 weeks	2	00
Last 6 months, 15-minute appointments, every 4 weeks	1	30
	8	00

CASE HISTORY 4: EXCESSIVE HAIR ASSOCIATED WITH THYROID ABNORMALITY

Consultation

An older client, extremely overweight, is referred by a doctor for help with her excessive hair growth. The client has suffered for ten years from undersecretion of the thyroid gland, and is now on a course of controlling drugs for her systemic condition. This condition is considered to be the source of the hair problem. In addition, the client suffers from angina pectoris, which is possibly aggravated by her weight problem. The hair condition is an extensive growth, covering the area from the front of the ears, across the cheeks, upper lip, chin and throat. The hairs are very strong and horny, translucent or white in colour, and the follicles are completely filled by the abnormal tissue sheaths in many cases.

The skin is fortunately in excellent condition as the client has not interfered with the hairs in any way apart from cutting them off occasionally to tidy herself up. Medical approval has been given for the treatment, with the proviso that when the client does not feel equal to epilation treatment, she must postpone her appointments. Since she suffers from both a thyroid and a heart complaint, it is inevitable that she will have good and bad periods, and the treatment must be adjusted accordingly. Low levels of current are recommended, applied with fairly long pauses between individual probes, to allow the client to cope with the sensation without anxiety or stress on the heart.

Treatment Plan

As the client is an older woman and has become adjusted over the years to her hirsute appearance, it is unlikely that she will be tempted to remove the hairs during her treatment programme, apart from occasional cutting. Any improvement will be appreciated by her. Discussion reveals that she most dislikes the hairs growing from small moles, as well as those growing along the jaw-line which are curly and occasionally become impacted. (Impacted hairs are hairs which are curled around themselves within the follicle and cause a small, septic, boil-like spot as they emerge onto the surface.)

Treatment is given in thirty minute sessions, using the low-slow method (roughly equivalent to twenty minutes of normal epilation), with appointments once a week, and work taking place on different areas on each occasion. The needle used is a .004 diameter Ferrie needle, and the intensity 2½ to 3½ depending on the hair strength, with the quantity of current applied controlled on the finger button. As the problem is so immense this amount of treatment will not bring about any quick improvement, but it fits the client's finances and her capacity for treatment.

Treatment Progression

Treatment is begun by removing the most obvious, long, curly hairs growing from tiny fibrous growths, and this quickly improves the client's general appearance. As the client's heart condition reduces her capacity for current intensity, only a part of each treatment time can be spent on these strong hairs, and this work must be interspersed with treatment of the more general growth on the face. The hairs on the lip, cheek and chin areas are also exceptionally strong and keratinized, and application has to be undertaken very carefully to achieve follicle entry because the follicles are filled with the hairs' outer sheaths. (This overgrowth of the tissue sheath appears to be present whenever the increased hair growth is caused by some abnormality of the endocrine system.)

The first complete removal of all the original hairs takes approximately eighteen months, mainly because treatment has been irregular due to fluctuations in the client's health. Bearing in mind the density of the hairs and their strength, this is a satisfactory achievement. Work concentrated on removing all the hairs at least once to reduce their strength, rather than attempting to clear any one area. By this stage, then, most of the hairs are finer and less distorted, and the skin is more settled. No more impacted hairs are growing, and the treatment has become more normal and easier to complete, and, therefore, progress is faster.

Surprisingly, the client's regrowth rate is very low, and any regrowth hairs which do occur because of the low current intensity are much finer than would be normal for hairs of this diameter. Reasons for this are hard to determine, thus underlining the difficulty of prognosis or assessment of how long a hair condition may take to resolve. The lack of previous interference with the hairs could be a contributory factor. Or, perhaps the client had no real predisposition to the hypertrichosis, the hair growth being instigated entirely by her physical condition, and once the health problem was brought under control, the stimulus for the hair growth was curtailed, leaving the client with a hair problem which did not regress or disappear.

After eighteen months of continuous treatment the appointments now become fortnightly, although still of thirty minutes' duration. The growth is now mainly finer, regrowth hair, and current intensity can be lowered, allowing more removals to be completed at each appointment. Results come quickly from this stage onwards with entire areas beginning to clear—first the cheeks downwards, below the eyes, emerge free from hair. Work on the lip hairs continues at a reduced current intensity, and applications begin on the difficult hairs on the throat, which are angled pointing downwards. The treatment is by now more general, with removals being accomplished in all areas where hairs remain. Systematically the hairs growing in concentrated clumps are removed, by degrees, until these areas are also less dense. The clumps on either side of the chin are always the most difficult to clear because of the concentration of current in a small area, which necessitates long healing gaps before further treatment can be applied.

Within two years the client has reached the stage of presenting a neat appearance to the world. Monthly appointments will suffice to clear the remaining hairs. Increased interest in her appearance has resulted in improved efforts to control her weight and follow more diligently her medically prescribed diet. The client looks younger and trimmer, and is delighted with the overall result of the treatment.

Tidy-up appointments at three-monthly intervals to keep the client neat and check progress becomes the final stage of the treatment plan.

Treatment Application	Total Treatment Time	
	Hours	Minutes
First 18 months, 30-minute appointments, weekly	36	00
Next 6 months, 30-minute appointments, fortnightly	6	00
Next 6 months, 30-minute appointments, monthly	3	00
	45	00

Plus tidy-up appointments—every three months, or longer.

CASE HISTORY 5: HAIR CONDITION RESULTING FROM HORMONE REPLACEMENT THERAPY (HRT)

Consultation

A very fashion-conscious, young, married woman, looking much younger than her thirty-five years, has a noticeable hair growth problem affecting the upper lip, and, to a lesser extent, the chin. The lip hairs are very fine, shallowly placed in the skin, and made more obvious by the client's natural, dark colouring. Hairs on the chin are stronger, spaced out, but more deeply placed in the skin. The skin is rather sensitive, and the client a rather tense, highly strung person. The hair growth can be directly traced to hormone replacement therapy following a total hysterectomy four years earlier. Lack of female hormones caused by the removal of the ovaries as well as the womb resulted in tiredness, lack of energy and sexual drive, and this has been remedied by a tiny hormone implant, placed into the superficial tissues of the lower abdominal area (bikini line). The implant has to be replaced approximately every twelve to eighteen months in this case, the exact length of time depending on the client's state of health. With the necessity of maintaining this level of artificial hormones, the hair problem is likely to become worse rather than better, and progress might be slow. Medical approval has been given for the epilation treatment.

Treatment Plan

Due to the client's skin sensitivity and low pain threshold, as well as her desire to maintain a groomed appearance, work must progress slowly. Being a hairdresser, the client understands the need to tackle the problem correctly, and is conscientious about keeping regular appointments. The treatment plan seeks to gain the best results as quickly as possible by giving ten minute appointments every ten days.

Treatment Progression

Skin reaction is initially severe, but skin healing is excellent. Rest gaps between appointments are built into the programme periodically to give the skin a chance to recover, and during these periods the client removes the hairs by cutting them off close to the surface. As the lip hairs are very fine in texture and emerge from minute follicles, while being shallowly placed in the skin, they are treated using a .003 Ferrie needle. The hairs prove to be more stubborn than their size would indicate, possibly due to hormonal stimulus, and have strong root structures. The skin's sensitivity and client's discomfort limit the amount of intensity that can be used, and in ten minutes of treatment the entire lip area is red and unable to cope with more treatment. Cool, ozone vapour steaming is used initially to reduce the reaction. However, it has subsequently been realized that the strong reaction flared quickly, but disappeared almost as rapidly, and was really due to anxiety over the treatment. As the tension over the treatment lessens, so does this reaction, and treatment can settle down. The client's determination to resolve this flaw in her looks keeps her attending regularly for treatment, even though she finds it really painful, despite a current intensity level of only 1 to 1½.

Regrowth is worse than normal for hairs of this diameter, and this point is discussed with the client to encourage her in the perseverance needed to get past this uphill and difficult stage in the treatment plan. After four months of conscientious attendance, this is accomplished, and progress improves, with regrowth hairs still proving a problem but reducing slowly, and areas of the lip becoming clear of hairs. The entire area of the upper lip has been treated equally, with hairs in the painful area under the nose being dealt with a few at a time in conjunction with treatment in other areas. This is done in order to prevent them being treated all a once, a situation which would prove unbearable for the client. Operators sometimes have to be a little devious about this point when treating nervous clients, and slip in a few of the more painful removals on 'good' days when the clients seem able to cope with more discomfort than usual. This balances up 'bad' days, when very little is achieved or when the treatment has to be concluded prematurely because the client is exceptionally tense or feeling the epilation badly for some reason.

By seven months, the problem is resolved almost entirely, and following a one month holiday break, which is used to rest the skin, treatment restarts at a slower rate, with monthly appointments to clear and tidy. After this, appointments are given every three to six weeks, depending on the hormone replacement therapy treatment. An upsurge in hair growth from different follicles is apparent when the implant is replaced, and for this reason the long, downy growth apparent on the cheeks and chin is also treated to remove its capacity for growth before it starts.

Treatment Application	Total Treatment Time	
	Hours	Minutes
First 3 months, 10-minute appointments, 10 days apart	1	30
Next month, rest—no treatment		
Next 3 months, 10-minute appointments, 10 days apart	1	30
Next month, rest—no treatment		
Next 3 months, 15-minute appointments, one month apart		45
Next 3 months, 15-minute appointments, 6 weeks apart		30
Next 3 months, 15-minute appointments, 3 weeks apart (implant replaced)	1	00
	5	15

Plus tidy-up treatments when needed.

CASE HISTORY 6: BREAST HAIR CONDITION LINKED WITH THE PILL

Consultation

A young client of French/Armenian extraction, recently married, has a breast hair problem which has arisen after she started taking the Pill in the early days of her marriage. She has now changed to a low dosage Pill, and indicates that she will be using this as her form of contraception for another year prior to starting a family. The hair growth is fine, very dense and dark and covers the area between the breasts, the inside area of each breast and around the nipples. The nipple hairs are stronger than the general growth. Due to the client's slim build, very little flesh covers the breastbone area, and treatment here is likely to be painful. In the case of the nipple hairs, this lack of flesh makes treatment much easier to complete, as skin handling is easier to control.

Treatment Plan

As the client lives some distance away, appointments varying from thirty to fifty-five minutes in length are given whenever she can attend the clinic. By spacing out the work carefully and allowing short, momentary pauses between applications, the whole area can be treated in one session, and, where the hairs are well spaced entire sections can be completely cleared of hairs. The client's pain capacity is the limiting factor in the treatment rather than the skin, which, being dark and well balanced, stands up to the epilation very well. Hairs growing in the most painful areas or too closely spaced, must be worked on alternately, treating some and leaving others, to avoid converging heat reactions or client distress. Applications are given with an insulated steel needle, using a current intensity level of 2 on the breast hairs and 3 to 4 on the nipple hairs.

Treatment Progression

After several sessions and initial removal of all the hairs, a rest period of a month is given to allow regrowth to emerge. Regrowth can take anywhere from three to eight weeks to form, and the speed of regrowth will tell the operator much about the hormonal stimulation of the follicle and provide guidance as to the extent of the hair growth problem. For instance excessively fast regrowth indicates that the problem is likely to be rather difficult to resolve, and the emergence of new hairs in areas not previously involved also points to internal stimuli being at work. Since the client knows her own condition intimately, she is the best person to advise the operator of changes which occur in the growth pattern.

In this case, the hairs re-emerge within three weeks, indicating that the client is really susceptible to the hormonal changes in the body brought about by the use of the Pill. A certain racial predisposition is also evident, as shown by a fine but noticeable growth of hair on her upper lip, which does not appear to worry the client, and is not treated.

Treatment progresses on a periodic basis and after six months all the hairs have been removed twice and are at last regrowing in a paler, finer form. From this stage onwards improvement is rapid, and after two more monthly appointments, the regrowth hair becomes very isolated in nature.

Ten months later, a final, tidy-up appointment is given to treat both the isolated hairs and the wispy growth to prevent any recurrence. The client is no longer taking the Pill and hopes to start her family shortly.

Subsequently, the client became pregnant and did not experience any increase in hair growth at the onset of her pregnancy, a point about which she was delighted.

Treatment Application	*Total Treatment Time*	
	Hours	Minutes
Initial appointment, 45 minutes		45
Next appointment, one month later, 45 minutes		45
Next appointment, 3 weeks later, 45 minutes		45
Next month, rest period (for regrowth to emerge)		
Next appointment, 45 minutes (to clear regrowth partially)		45
Next appointment, 3 weeks later, 45 minutes (to clear regrowth)		45
Next appointment, 3 months later, 45 minutes (to clear stragglers)		45
10 months later, tidy-up and concluding session of 30 minutes		30
	5	00

CASE HISTORY 7:
GENERAL HIRSUTENESS
(FACIAL AND EYEBROW
EPILATION)

Consultation

An active lady in her mid-forties who has always suffered from a hair problem finds it has worsened in her middle years. The condition has reached a stage where she has a severe upper-lip and chin problem of exceptionally strong hairs, heavy, hairy brows and isolated, long hairs on the cheeks and in front of her ears. Her appearance is one of a really hairy woman. The client is a natural red-head, with a strong curl to her hair. The superfluous hairs are horny, translucent or white in colour, and have abnormally deep roots and long follicles. The tissues sheaths fill the follicles, making needle entry very difficult, and, in addition, the skin is very florid and reacts strongly to the epilation treatment. The client previously plucked the hairs, until they became too strong, and then chemical depilatories were used. As the problem is going to take a long time to resolve, a plan is devised to treat the worst areas first.

Treatment Plan

Treatment initially concentrates on removing the more isolated of the most untidy hairs on the chin and cheeks, and starting work on the upper lip, where the growth is very strong and closely spaced, with a concentration of hairs under the nose. The treatment plan is to work a little on each area at each appointment, thereby helping the skin to cope with the effects of the diathermy current, while making continuous forward progress. Skin reactions are extreme, but fade quickly. The client suffers very little scabbing or blood spotting, which might have been expected with the extreme strength of the hairs. Several needle diameters are used, as the growth is very varied, but the removals are mainly accomplished using a .004 Ferrie steel needle. A moderate current intensity level is found to cause the least skin reaction and to be the most bearable for the client. Current intensity varies from 2½ to 6, according to the hair growth and its location, and adjustments are mainly made by the button tap or foot-switch.

This client stands her periods of treatment very well and heals rapidly. Thirty minute appointments are booked on a fortnightly basis, with the work being of general nature, and covering all areas.

Treatment Progression

For the first few months of treatment, the facial growth is very untidy and the skin looks rather disturbed. As all areas are being treated at the same time, it is difficult for the client to tidy up her appearance by temporary methods without slowing the progress of the epilation. The hairs are cut, but as they grow so rapidly they are always visible for treatment.

At one appointment, the skin became too red to continue treatment in the usual areas, and so a few very long, straggly hairs were removed from the eyebrows. This has improved their appearance so much that the client has decided to have them reshaped by continuing the treatment. Although it is preferable to split facial and brow work into two appointments, the client prefers to have all her work completed at the one visit. As she is a working woman and her time is at a premium, and as her personal tolerance for epilation is very good, this is agreed upon and appointments are extended to forty-five minutes.

The brows are excessively hairy, and at first it is simply a question of thinning out the bulk of the hairs and removing the long, horny hairs which grow out at all angles. A smoother, fine brow is aimed for, and the work is carried out evenly on both brows until the final shape emerges.

After eight months of treatment, the original hairs have regrown in a form which is easier to treat, quicker to remove and requires less current intensity. The brows are beginning to look like eyebrows rather than just a mass of hair, and the entire appearance looks lighter and less hirsute. The client is very pleased with the progress, and eager to complete the treatment, so fortnightly appointments continue. Because the problem is so generalized, it takes eighteen months to overcome the worst of the problem, despite a remarkable treatment capacity, good healing ability and a very stoical attitude to the whole treatment on the part of the client.

At the end of two years, this very dear lady is much improved in appearance. Her brows and the centre of the upper-lip area are the only parts still causing a real problem, and this is mainly because the hairs here are so numerous and in such a tiny area that, to avoid over-reaction, treatment must be well-spaced. In addition, work in this area causes watering of the eyes and sneezing which, added to the extreme discomfort of the lip work, makes progress rather slow. Because of the limited amount of work that can be applied to these localized areas, appointments are reduced in length, although kept at fortnightly intervals.

It is decided to rest the lip area for a few weeks and give the skin a real chance to recover, while concentrating on the brow hairs. The client has decided that, as her looks are so improved, she will have a few fibrous growths removed from her neck, and this is completed satisfactorily.

Clients often become much more interested in their appearance after they have overcome a really severe hair problem, and many times go on to undertake further treatment to complete their groomed appearance, such as reshaping brows, removing naevi, or even moving on to another area altogether, such as removing leg hairs. In the case of really hirsute individuals, however, some compromise has to be sought; although they would love to be hair-free, this is really not possible. The operator must use her judgement in advising the client on the best results that can be achieved with the money and time available.

At the end of two and a half years, the problem is almost resolved, and work proceeds slowly on the brows and lip. Appointments continue every two months for two more years, then every three months and finally six-monthly intervals. The tendency to hypertrichosis cannot be cured, but it has been controlled, and further hair growth can be removed at the periodic tidy-up appointments.

Treatment Application	*Total Treatment Time*	
	Hours	Minutes
First 4 months, 30-minute appointments, fortnightly	4	00
Next 4 months, 45-minute appointments, fortnightly	6	00
Next 10 months, 45-minute appointments, fortnightly	15	00
Next 6 months, 45-minute appointments, fortnightly	9	00
Next 6 months, 30-minute appointments, fortnightly	6	00
Next 6 months, 30-minute appointments, 2-monthly	1	30
Next 6 months, 30-minute appointments, 3-monthly	1	00
	42	30

Plus 6 monthly tidying appointments, or as needed.

CASE HISTORY 8:
BEARD HAIR GROWTH
ON A TRANSSEXUAL
(SEX-CHANGE PATIENT)

Consultation

An adult has been recommended for treatment to remove hair growth on the beard area following a sex change operation from male to female. The client is still taking feminizing hormones to improve her appearance, grow breasts, and hopefully reduce hair growth in the male sexual pattern. She is also still undergoing psychotherapy to help her readjust to her new female role in life, following years of unhappiness as a natural, if ill-suited, male.

The beard hair remains in its original form and needs long-term treatment. The strong, dark hairs are removed by daily shaving, and the 'four o'clock shadow' is hidden by make-up. The skin is in good condition, and medical approval is given for the treatment, although the electrologist is advised that the patient is emotionally unstable and temperamental and unlikely to be an ideal client. The evidence is that few sex-change patients ever complete their treatment programme or resolve their hair problem.

Treatment Plan

As the area to be treated is extensive, daily shaving will remain a necessity into the foreseeable future, but the areas of the throat and cheeks which are going to be treated will have to be allowed to grow. These areas will require camouflaging with creams or make-up, according to the client's preference.

As most of the hairs are strong, being normal secondary hairs in the male pattern, the applications must be well spaced, and all the treatment areas covered in a chequered fashion. Hairs emerging in small clumps are treated by removing one hair and leaving the others for later sessions. Treatment sessions are thirty minutes in length, and, as the problem is so vast, different areas are treated in rotation—lip and chin, or cheeks and throat, etc. Appointments are booked as and when the client's time and finances allow. Transsexual patients are erratic, unsettled individuals who seldom fit into a regular appointment pattern, and, therefore, the electrologist must be prepared to be available for treatment at the client's convenience. Early evening appointments are usually preferred as this avoids the necessity of meeting other clients. However, such clients are usually much embarrassed by their appearance, and are often prepared to devote a lot of time and money to improve it.

In this case, the hairs are all very similar in diameter, and a strong current intensity is needed to remove them. The client finds the 'high-fast' method of treatment most bearable, and this is applied using .004 and .005 diameter Ferrie needles and intensity levels ranging from 3½ to 7, controlled by very short application taps. Appointments are twice weekly on average, and the client copes very well with the treatment, although she finds it hard to admit that the problem is any more severe than any other woman's. Such self-delusion is often the reason for failure to carry through the treatment programme; results are expected far sooner than is possible, and the clients get depressed about their progress.

Treatment Progression

Twice-weekly appointments continue for eighteen months, by which time most of the original hairs have been removed once, or in many cases twice, and mainly regrowth hair is being treated. The results are helped by the administration of the controlling hormonal drugs which reduce regrowth from the treated follicles.

Two years after starting treatment, the client can manage without shaving, simply cutting emerging hairs close to the skin. The strength of the hairs has been reduced, and they are present in a finer, paler form as long, wispy hairs.

Six months later, the client presents a reasonably clear skin, and only one appointment a week is needed to conclude the treatment. Eventually, these appointments become three-monthly, and finally the client comes for help only when it is needed. She has overcome one of the major problems of changing sex.

Very few transsexual patients have this degree of determination, and often give up just as they are beginning to win through against the hair condition. Electrologists must be very patient with these individuals if they decide to undertake treatment outside the hospital situation. They must be made to understand that the operator is willing to offer help when it is needed and understands their special problems.

Treatment Application	Total Treatment Time	
	Hours	Minutes
First 18 months, 30-minute appointments, twice-weekly (rather irregular)	70	00
Next 6 months, 30-minute appointments, twice-weekly	24	00
Next 6 months, 30-minute appointments, twice-weekly (rather irregular)	15	00
Next 6 months, 30-minute appointments, weekly (rather irregular in patches)	8	00
Next 6 months, 30-minute appointments, 3-monthly	1	00
	118	00

Plus additional sessions when needed.

CASE HISTORY 9: EXCESSIVE HAIR GROWTH DUE TO HEREDITARY FACTORS

Consultation

An attractive young woman, twenty years of age, has excessive hair growth on the chin and isolated, strong hairs on the cheeks and neck. The chin growth requires daily shaving, and the young woman hesitated before seeking help because she realized that, once treatment commenced, her secret would be revealed. She had taken the courage to tell her boyfriend about her problem, and, with his support, has now decided to seek help.

The hairs are horny and keratinized, and initially prove very difficult to remove as they fill the follicle entirely; they have in fact, caused the natural follicle size to become distended, leaving open pores on removal of the hairs. So, it is important to use the finest needles possible in order not to worsen this problem of increased pore size, and also to minimize the pain element in the treatment.

The hairs are present as a result of a hereditary factor—the problem had been present in a great-grandmother, but had skipped two generations to turn up again with the young client. Medical advice had been sought, and epilation suggested as the best form of treatment.

The client is soon to be married and has started taking the Pill. This may prove an added complication, by restricting the possible progress of the treatment. However, a plan has been devised to provide treatment, while maintaining as immaculate an appearance as possible. Treatments are booked for Mondays so that sufficient hairs will grow over the weekend to a length that can be treated. Fortunately, the client has not previously used hair removal treatments such as waxing or chemical depilatories, but has coped by daily shaving and heavy camouflaging make-up to get her through each day.

So, all the hairs are present, and the client proves to be a very brave young woman, excellent in the treatment situation, with few reactions to the applications and with a very co-operative attitude to resolving her long-term problem. The length of treatment is discussed, and a lot of encouragement given about the *permanence* of epilation, to balance the cost and time involved in gaining a final, hair-free facial appearance.

Treatment Plan

The treatment is applied in a well-spaced manner, all over the affected area, using a fine insulated needle to keep down skin reaction. A rounded, probe end .004 diameter needle is used to apply a current intensity of 3½ to 4, with excellent results. Other finer needles (possibly down to .003) will probably be used to treat finer regrowth hair, as this helps to reduce discomfort. The probes must be undertaken very carefully because many of the hairs are distorted in nature, having thick sheaths and being of a very horny texture.

Skin reaction is initially fierce and care is taken in the use of soothing lotions and the usual pre- and aftercare measures. However, it settles down as treatment progresses and the client becomes accustomed to the diathermy current. Healing seems excellent, and the client is advised to take special care with her health to assist in the healing process.

A high level of intensity, applied for a fraction of a second, proves to be most bearable for the client and results in the easiest removals. However, great care must be taken to avoid current transference due to needle movement. For this reason, applications are slow but accurate, especially at the first appointment to help the client to adjust to the discomfort involved.

Treatment Progression

In order to get well ahead with the treatment plan, both to encourage the client and to improve her appearance quickly because of the imminent wedding date, weekly appointments are made, taking care to treat only those areas not previously treated until healing is complete. The skin heals very well, and within a month considerable improvement has been made.

The treatment plan makes allowance for shaving, as long as enough hairs of adequate length for treatment are left when the appointment day arrives. Excellent co-operation on this point enables good, fast results to be achieved and six months after her wedding, the hairs have cleared and thinned down sufficiently for the client to manage almost without the need to shave daily. Appointments are now every two weeks, and more work can be accomplished during each twenty minute session, as many hairs are of the regrowth type. Excessive regrowth has not occurred as the client had not interfered with the hairs other than simply cutting them off at the surface by shaving.

Within one year, the problem is well under control. All the isolated hairs on the cheeks and neck have gone, and the areas of more concentrated growth, where the skin itself restricted the amount of current used, are now all regrowth hairs and no longer a disfigurement. The treatment intervals are now extended to three weeks, to help prevent dehydration and loss of skin texture which is associated with over-treatment.

Within eighteen months the problem is resolved. The actual number of treatment hours has not been excessive and the skin is still in a good condition. In this case, taking the Pill does not seem to have caused any undue delay in the progress of the treatment, although, naturally, one cannot be sure. As the background to the hypertrichosis is genetic, all the hairs are removed, leaving only the very finest vellus growth. This is done to avoid the risk of an increased hair growth problem resulting from either a pregnancy with its associated high hormone levels or the continued use of the Pill over a number of years. The increased growth may not show itself for many years, as we saw earlier, but individuals genetically disposed to excessive hair growth, are always at risk and, therefore, the safest thing is to remove the follicles' capacity to even sustain a normal fine hair, making its growth potential very poor, and so less susceptible to hormonal stimulus from within.

Treatment Application	Total Treatment Time	
	Hours	Minutes
First 2 months, 20-minute appointments, weekly	2	40
Break of one month (pre-wedding and honeymoon)		
Next 3 months, 20-minute appointments, weekly	4	00
Next 6 months, 20-minute appointments, fortnightly	4	00
Next 6 months, 20-minute appointments, 3-weekly	2	40
	13	20

Tidy-up treatments given as and when needed.

Useful Addresses

**PROFESSIONAL
ORGANIZATIONS AND
EXAMINATION BOARDS**

Further information on courses is available from the following examination boards and professional organizations:

American Electrolysis Association
710 Tennent Road, Englishtown, NJ 07726, USA

Beauty Therapy Club by Ann Gallant
Esthetic and Beauty Supply, 180 Bentley Street, Markham, Ontario, Canada L3R 3L2

E. A. Ellisons & Co Ltd, Brindley Road South, Exhall, Coventry CV7 9EP, UK

British Association of Beauty Therapy and Cosmetology
Secretary Mrs D. Parkes, Suite 5, Wolesley House, Oriel Road, Cheltenham GL50 1TH, UK

British Association of Electrolysis
6 Quakers Mede, Haddenham, Bucks HP17 8EB, UK

British Biosthetic Society
2 Birkdale Drive, Bury, Greater Manchester BL8 2SG, UK

City and Guilds of London Institute
46 Britannia Street, London WC1 9RG, UK

Le Comité Internationale D'Esthétiques et de Cosmetologie, (CIDESCO)
CIDESCO International Secretariat, PO Box 9, A1095 Vienna, Austria

Confederation of Beauty Therapy and Cosmetology
Education Secretary Mrs B. Longhurst, 3 The Retreat, Lidwells Lane, Goudhurst, Kent, UK

Electrolysis Association of Ontario
Box 287, Thornhill, Ontario, Canada L3T 3N3

Institute of Electrolysis
251 Seymour Grove, Manchester M16 0DS, UK

International Guild of Professional Electrologists
3209 Premier Drive, Suite 124, Plano, TX 75075, USA

International Health and Beauty Council, (IHBC)
PO Box 36, Arundel, West Sussex BN18 0SW, UK

International Therapy Examination Centre, (ITEC)
50 Queen Street, Henley-on-Thames, Oxon, UK
The Northern Institute of Massage
100 Waterloo road, Blackpool FY4 1AW, UK
Skin Care Association of America
16 West 57th Street, New York, NY, USA
South African Institute of Health and Beauty Therapists
PO Box 56318, Pinegowrie 2123, South Africa
United Professional Electrolysis Manufacturers Association (UPEMA)
49 Arnold Street, Riverside, RI 02915, USA

EQUIPMENT MANUFACTURERS

Ann Gallant Beauté Therapy Equipment
Esthetic and Beauty Supply, 180 Bentley Street, Markham, Ontario, Canada L3R 3L2
Tel: 416 479 2929 Fax (416) 479 7303
Beauty Gallery Equipment by Ann Gallant
E. A. Ellisons & Co Ltd, Brindley Road South, Exhall, Coventry CV7 9EP, UK
Clare Inc.
13026 San Fernando Road, Sylmar, CA 91342, USA
Depilex Ltd and **Slimaster Beauty Equipment Ltd**
Regent House, Dock Road, Birkenhead, Merseyside L41 1DG, UK
E. A. Ellisons & Co Ltd
Brindley Road South, Exhall, Coventry CV7 9EP, UK
Fischer Co. Inc.
517 Commercial Street, Glendale, CA 91203, USA
George Solley Organization Ltd
James House, Queen Street, Henley on Thames, Oxon, UK
Instantron Company
3124 Pawtucket Avenue, East Providence, Rhode Island, USA
Interscan Solarium
61 Balmoral Road, Gillingham, Kent ME7 1BR, UK
Nemectron Belmont Inc
17 West 56th Street, New York, NY 10019, USA
Proteus Inc.
PO Box 211, Bellingham, MA 02019, USA
Silhouette International Beauty Equipment
Kenwood Road, Reddish, Stockport, Cheshire SK5 6PH, UK

Slendertone Ltd
12–14 Baker Street, London W1M 2HA, UK
Sudonna Inc.
41 Bergenline Avenue, Westwood, NJ 07675, USA
Taylor Reeson Ltd
96–98 Dominion Road, Worthing, Sussex, UK

TREATMENT PRODUCT SUPPLIERS

E. A. Ellisons & Co Ltd
(Bulk and specialized treatment suppliers)
Brindley Road, Exhall, Coventry CV7 9EP, UK
Elizabeth of Schwarzenberg
113 Guildford Street, Chertsey, Surrey KT16 9AS, UK
Clarins (UK) Ltd
(Oils and body products)
150 High Street, Stratford, London E15 2NE, UK
Ann Gallant Beauté Therapy Products
Ann Gallant Clinic Supplies
Skin Care, Treatment and Specialized Products for the professional operator (Facial, Body, Electrology) from E. A. Ellisons & Co Ltd, Brindley Road South, Exhall, Coventry CV7 9EP, UK
Pier Augré Cosmetics
Harbourne Marketing Associates, Oak House, 271 Kingston Road, Leatherhead, Surrey, UK
Thalgo Cosmetic/Importex
(Marine based products)
5 Tristan Square, Blackheath, London SE3 9UB, UK

SOURCES OF EMPLOYMENT AND PRIVATE TRAINING

Seligman & Latz Inc, 'ESSANELLE'
Executive Offices:
International Division,
6 Curzon Place, London W1, UK;
Head Office:
666 Fifth Avenue, New York, NY, USA
The Tao Clinic
Head Office:
153 Brompton Road, London SW3, UK

BEAUTY CLUB

ESTHETIC AND BEAUTY SUPPLY
180 Bentley Street,
Markham, Ontario, Canada L3R 3L2
Tel: 416 479 2929

E. A. ELLISONS & CO. LTD.
Brindley Road South,
Exhall,
Coventry CV7 9EP, UK
Tel: 0203 362505

WHAT DOES *CLUB* MEMBERSHIP OFFER YOU?

— A feeling of belonging to a truly international club.
— Regular BEAUTY CLUB newsheets to support this linked-in Club feeling
— The right to wear the BEAUTY CLUB badge, which shows your interest in the Beauty World
— BEAUTY CLUB Members Card for preferential buyers term
— Information and expertise from leading experts in the field
— News of latest advances in the industry
— Technical fact sheets for fast easy reference on products, equipment, and treatment systems, etc.
— Buying discounts on a wide range of goods, using your BEAUTY CLUB Card
— A chance to take advantage of 'SPECIAL OFFERS' on the latest and best in the business
— A link into Beauty Education International for:
   Books, Beauty Guides, Technical Information, Research & Development Programmes, Clinic Planning Guidance, Equipment Design, and Post Graduate Training Courses

WHO CAN JOIN THE *BEAUTY CLUB*?

Anyone who is interested in the Beauty Industry, and wants to keep up to date and in touch with the latest knowledge and tech niques available to help them in their work.

A. GALLANT
F.S.H.B.Th., Int.B.Th.Dip, D.R.E

BEAUTY EDUCATION INTERNATIONAL

Beauty Club at
E. A. Ellisons & Co Ltd.
Brindley Road South,
Exhall,
Coventry CV7 9EP, UK
Tel: 0203 362505

An international organization whose aim is to raise the standards of beauty therapy by means of training, educational material, equipment information and supply, and management consultancy.

Its aim is to motivate, communicate, and educate within the beauty industry, through membership, newsletters, instructional material, books, tapes, and basic and postgraduate training information and supply.

Beauty Education International acts as a reference point for all those involved in beauty therapy and through their own club keeps them informed of all the latest developments in the industry around the world.

Index

Main references are indicated by italic page numbers